Breasts Don't Lie

Trudi Young Taylor

*To Ron
A wonderful writer*

Copyright 2014 © Trudi Young Taylor
All rights reserved.

This book or any portion thereof may not be reproduced or used in any manner whatsoever without the express written permission of the author.

Interior design by Sable Books
Cover image by John Rowe

Sable Books
sablebooks.org

Preface

I finished the first draft of my first book and had the usual depressing thoughts of a writer. "This sucks. I have nothing else to say. I'm just exhausted."

My writing group let me wallow for precisely ten minutes and then said, "Get off your ass. Write something. Anything."

"But about what?" I said, piteously and horribly self-indulgent.

They looked around and then at the group's leader. She said, "Write about something you know."

Truly, at that point I couldn't think of anything more that I knew. I stared at the blank pages in front of me, thought about crying, and then I looked down. I thought, "These are my breasts. I know my breasts. I know about breasts." I giggled. "This could be a fun writing exercise. I'm sure I have stuff to get off my chest, so to speak."

The next week, I returned to the writing group with a short-short story about the temptation of a buttered, honey soaked biscuit versus glorious, tasty mounds of breasts. The other writers talked and talked and talked about the story. I had an epiphany – not only are there few places where people get to talk about breasts, people like to talk about breasts, boobs, fun bubbles, or the girls.

Take a second and look at your breasts. All of you –

men and women. Do you really know your breasts? Do you know their anatomy? How do feel about them? Do you even pay any attention to them? Do other people pay attention to them? Do you look away? Your breasts are awesome and an important part of you. And they impact other important components of your lives, your body image, your sexuality, your fears and desires, your individual story, and the stories of your family and culture. I guarantee if we meet, you will look at my breasts. And that's okay until I say it isn't. I know I will glance at yours.

Writing this book has made it okay for me to acknowledge my own breasts, their history, and to see your breasts. It has made talking about breasts less embarrassing and even fun. Our breasts have histories influenced by culture, biology, genetics, medicine, and the fashion industry. Reading this book could be a catalyst for you to come to grips, literally and metaphorically, with your breasts and the myriad of breasts around you in a respectful, reverent, even playful way.

This book contains a series of short stories running from a few pages to many pages. The stories are fictionalized versions of people's adventures plus slightly altered tales from my fifty odd years on this planet. I have written most of the stories without detailed settings to allow the reader to project themselves into the stories. With some luck, they will trigger associations with personal, familial, relational, and cultural happenings. I am sure I have left out some important ideas, issues, and viewpoints, and I welcome you to contact me with your reactions and suggestions. This book is intended to spark dialogue and to be a work in progress. With your help, it can be.

The book's goal is to challenge your ideas and feelings – stir the pot enough to create a dialogue within you and with others. To facilitate this, at the end of each story is a summary of information arising from the theme of the story, references, a series of exercises, and a resource section. The stories are arranged by life decades but they can be read in any order. Hopefully, you can use the book in classrooms, support groups, and book clubs. The goal is to get you talking about and developing compassion for this subject, near and dear to your heart.

After writing the first story, I sent out an email to my friends asking for personal recollections about breasts: how they felt about their breasts and the breasts of their partners. Brave friends volunteered anecdotes, delightful and troubling. Men and women talked openly to me about their squeamishness and discomfort over the changes in their lovers' health and appearance. I spent a lot of time looking in the mirror at my own breasts - equally marveling and feeling dismayed by the changes brought on by time and medical procedures. Common experiences and exceptional snippets became the plots and themes for most of the stories.

People were generous and truthful. One man was comfortable enough over morning coffee to say, "I like big floppy ones that I can wear like ear muffs." Apart from the mind-ripping mental image of my friend as a lover, as a person who evaluated breasts for their ... floppiness, the statement forced me to begin responding to him as a complete man, really smart, funny, honest, and sexual. Then he made my heart sing. He told me how he had discussed it with his wife, admittedly "not floppy," before they were married. How many of us discuss these issues with our lovers? I pledged right away to be more open with all potential lovers. I may have gone a bit overboard.

Some research was done on the Internet through different medical groups, associations for information/support/education, and consulting with medical specialists of multiple disciplines. Surprisingly, when I Googled books about breasts, the available books were either pornographic or medical. For such an interesting topic, there was a dearth of books to help people talk about their experiences and feelings around this universal body part. Many women and one man talked with truth and pain about the long-term consequences of having undergone treatment for cancer. I talked to people about their experiences with the medical community and even went to three breast surgeons to see what that was like. I talked to the surgeons and their nurses about their personal responses to their patients' procedures. I fell in love with the good-looking plastic surgeon who said to me, "Breasts. Men are just happy to see them. Never mind, touch them."

But I still wondered, after all this talking and encouragement, if there was enough substance to merit writing a book about breasts. I had the nerve wrenching opportunity to present two stories at open reading nights. On the first occasion, I received raucous applause. It wasn't until later I realized that my strapless dress was covered by the podium, and I therefore looked naked as I read about men's responses to nipples. It taught me to pay more attention to my presentation – of my breasts. I left the reading elated by the responses of the men in the audience. I had touched a nerve with them. They wanted to talk and laugh about their own ambivalence over men and women's breasts. On another occasion, my reading ended in polite clapping. People were distressed by the story's subject matter - lovers dealing with an upcoming surgery. To my audiences, I am grateful for the chance to read and to receive feedback from you.

Throughout the four-year journey, my writing group has been wonderfully supportive. In many ways, the book is a group effort at understanding and support. Over some stories we agreed and over other stories, we had long heated discussions, thereby fulfilling the book's purpose!

To all these people, I want to say, "Your honesty was wonderful. Without it, the book would not exist. These stories are a tribute to you and your breasts." The little short story to get me back into writing has turned into a four-year adventure. I will never look at breasts, yours or mine, the same way, ever again. Thank you. Thank you. Thank you.

Trudi Taylor
December 5, 2013
Raleigh, NC

Contents:

List of stories

These stores were written to evoke memories and invite reflection on personal, familial, relational, and cultural issues. The stories are arranged into groupings by decade. Following each story is a discussion of the theme of the story with references, activities, and resources to help the reader explore beliefs, feelings, and behaviors. The stories can be read in chronological order or in any order that is compelling and relevant to them.

The Teens: Breast Buds—the beginning awareness of breasts in our world.

First Crop   1

The purchase of a first bra strengthens the bond between a mother and her sulky preteen daughter. Delicate daisies embroidered on yellow cotton initiates the twelve year old into womanhood and realigns roles in a matriarchy.

A Prehistoric Bug   19

Two adolescents explore personal responsibility through the high school halls of aching sexuality. What happens to us when we carry the label of "good girl," "good boy," or their opposites throughout our life?

The 20s: Breasts symbolize desirability and fertility.

Visual Coffee Breaks   35

Are breasts more nutritious, more tempting, or more fattening than a buttered, honey soaked biscuit? Lovers discuss seduction and weight gain during a lunchtime tryst.

Unforced Errors   47

Two men watch women playing tennis. Their ambivalence around desire and their own body images pricks awareness. The men cover up. Must men be aware of their own bodies in the same way and to the same intensity as women for the score to be "Love-All"?

No Lying   59

A woman's liminal moment is triggered by milk on her green silk blouse. Is the choice to breastfeed or not a choice made by the woman, dictated by societal pressure, defined by the workplace, or mandated by the legal system?

The 30s: Breasts keep the secrets of our souls.

A Wide Gap   71

On Skype, a pant-less radiologist pontificates on the difference between a wide and a narrow gap on the hundreds of mammograms he evaluates daily. His long distance partner is curious about how the celluloid images of breasts impact his lust for her.

The Origami of Heartache — 85

Before her breast biopsy, a husband's rejection of his wife and her subsequent failure to address his fear tears apart their marriage. "When do you tell the secrets of your soul when your body cannot lie," wonders the sales manager who helps her.

Renovation — 117

The interconnection of female body image, aging, and desirability are explored in a drawer of underwear. Is she going to put on a push-up, lined or gel-padded bra? Will she go for the brass ring and apply the stick-ons?

The 40s: Our breasts define reflect our relationship to aging and mortality.

The Rose Garden — 137

Armed with a Sharpie, a couple plans for changes in their physical and emotional lives after surgery. The harsh lines of her surgeon's cuts become the fiercely honest adornments of lovers growing back together.

A Collection of Forks — 161

The perfect bra allows a middle-aged woman to re-enter the dating world as an empowered figure. Her date is not amused.

Got Milk   183

Can you express delight and disappointment without objectifying a body area? When two women talk about breast-feeding and desire, their changing relationships to their breasts are revealed in their choice of names.

The 50s and beyond: The changing breast reflects the transitions in our gender roles and personal power.

Beans on a Bus   199

The aftereffects of chemotherapy are reframed into a humorous emotional bond after a bus ride to the Catskills. Body image and sexuality are profoundly impacted by surgery, chemotherapy, and radiation. How does a couple get back on track after the derailment of breast cancer?

Lord Almighty   225

A daughter decides to redefine her breasts and sexuality throwing her parents' marriage into scrutiny. When roles are no longer determined by chromosomal gender, the history of love determines their behaviors.

Malignancy   243

At an academic luncheon, gender, race, and power explode with a man's primal fears – betrayal by his friends, colleagues, and own body. Breasts not only define the woman but the man.

Breasts Don't Lie

First Crop

My mother took me to Marks & Spencer when it was time to buy my first bra. "This is where Princess Anne buys her underwear," she said.

I did the usual teenage thing, rolled my eyes, slumped my shoulders while dragging my feet and mumbling. "Oh, goody. That's just bloody wonderful. Underwear like Princess Anne's. Lovely. I thought we were getting me a school uniform?"

"Don't get smart with me. You're a young lady now."

I lifted my nose, sniffed loudly, trying to discriminate between the regretfully common and the more genteel garments of womanhood. Mother's long fingered, delicately gloved hand reached for mine. She pulled me through the length of the only department store in Edinburgh. She trotted me past the women's clothes with the psychedelic flowered dresses then zigzagged us through the mod blouses and miniskirts to a secluded corner of the store. My eyes stared frantically at the racks of foreign female objects. The damp woolen scents of the medieval city were replaced with the unfamiliar tang of polyester, elastic, and impending maturity. I stumbled through the maze knowing that my childhood expectations of school and life would soon be thrown out along with last year's uniforms and my undershirts.

With the flash of knowledge came embarrassment—I knew I was 'unacceptably' dressed in shapeless tartan trews (a child's Scottish trousers) and last term's school sweater. Determined to never give up I said, "I hate this pukey green sweater."

"It's hunter green," said my mother. "Your school's color and very precious to Scotland." She pushed my shoulders out of their slouch and rearranged the sweater on my lumpy frame. "Stand up straight. You're in seventh form. The standards are higher for girls in seventh form."

"I still hate this sweater."

"Your Granny knit this sweater for you. Do you hate your Granny?"

Well she had me there. I loved my Granny, my great grandmother. After the early death of my mother's mother and with the strength of the aunties, Granny had helped my mother make a graceful transition into adulthood. Small and dainty, Mother moved in pleated skirts and cashmere sweaters of soft green or plum. Her red hair curled long down her back. The genteel scent of lilies of the valley followed her into rooms. Perfume, lipstick and gloves were always spotless: the proper demeanor of a graduate from the ultimate British boarding school, St. Margaret's College for Young Ladies.

To the regret and disapproval of the family and probably the school, my mother gave up a career as an opera singer, learned to type, and married a minimally Christian ship captain. But, despite her marriage, everyday Mother wore a pair of jade earrings in St. Margaret's hunter green and hung her Star of David inside her sweater but next to her heart.

Now, I was going to St. Margaret's and in danger of becoming the next family and boarding school disappointment. I didn't see how even Granny could help me. Over the summer, I had felt myself start to shift. I was resentful and fascinated in equal parts. The family women had seen the changes. The beginning curves of a womanly body betrayed me. To my way of thinking, the suggestion of hips and tiny breasts cursed me. Just last year, my body was so flat that I could disappear under rumpled sheets, avoiding the grown-ups.

But the women of my family noticed more than the changes in my body, they saw the blush on my face. When my cousin had asked me if I found her husband attractive, as a sullen child-woman, I replied, "I guess, for an old guy, he's ... cute." The women's laughter shamed and silenced me. I couldn't stop my body from moving into their world but my mind tightened against them. I wanted to hide out longer in childhood.

Outside the store, the Scottish sky changed from day to night. The sunset gathered pinks, purples, and dark red. A fall drizzle washed the soot covered building of Old Town. Term was a week away from starting at St. Margaret's. Families were buying school uniforms after a summer of unconscious playing in mismatched hand-me-downs. Buying underwear, admitting I had the beginnings of breasts, was, for sure, the most humiliating start to school I'd ever encountered. Not that school was ever the love of my life.

St. Margaret's was dedicated to turning out predictable and pliant females by the end of thirteen years of deportment classes, field hockey, art appreciation, and religious observance. The proscribed uniform consisted of a white blouse, green and yellow striped tie, dark green tunic, sweater, and crested blazer. The school dictated 'young ladies' had to wear a special type of fully covering knickers of a heavy and scratchy material dyed to match our sweaters. All the inmates, our nickname for boarders, had to wear the regulation underwear.

"This is not the correct shade. It's forest green," said my mother measuring a pair of the knickers against my bottom.

"Mom, put those down." I squirmed away to put a table of underwear between us.

"How repressed you are," she said, folding them neatly and returning them to the stack. "When you go into eighth form, you'll get to wear twinsets and skirts."

"Will Granny knit my twinsets?"

"No, those will be fitted cashmere and make the most of your figure."

"I want Granny to make my sweaters. And I don't have a figure."

I put another table of regulation underpants between us. My mother had looked at me and I saw her soften.

"We still need to get your uniform. Let's get this over with and we can have some tea." She moved past the tables of knickers. I made a break for the elevators. Mom grabbed my arm. She shook her head. We stood side by side next to a wall of bras. I refused to look up.

"Can we have tea now?"

"No," and she appraised my body. "Hmm, I was right. You will need a bra."

"No. No, I don't," I said looking down at my fairly flat chest. "Mom, I still score points for the other team."

"Being bad at field hockey does not preclude a bra." My mother returned my shot with as much skill as she had shown during her time on St. Margaret's hockey field.

I ran for the goal. "Yeah, the St. Maggie's Novices. They're brutes. Smacking each other with hockey sticks. Yelling bad words … "

"Lower your voice."

"You want me to be just like that. Want to hear what they scream?"

"You know it's not like that. I want what's best for

you. Give it." I unclasped my Star of David on the delicate silver chain and put it in my mother's palm. Her fingers curled around mine in a moment of shared duplicity. During the school term, my mother substituted my Star of David necklace with the Ionic Cross of Scotland, the symbol of a Celtic truce with Christianity. She knew the cruelty of anti-Semitism in schools and department stores.

Mother turned to look through the stacks of bras while firmly grasping my hand. Her head swiveled between me and the assortment of bras. My bright red face examined the floor as I tried to make myself as small as possible. I noticed my shoes needed polishing. Mother did not let go of my hand. "Stop fidgeting," she commanded and moved me to a table further down the aisle. I blushed and blushed as we passed rows of old lady underwear, so unlike the lacy garments hanging in our flat.

Not ready to surrender, I picked up the biggest bra I could find. Waving it at my mother, I said, "Will I look like this one day?" Mother snatched the bra out of my hand and walked quietly to a row of pretty patterned bras, yellow with pale creamy daisies printed on them. Picking out an assortment of sizes, she pointed to the dressing room: a small closet with a badly fitting curtain. I shuffled towards it.

"Get a move on. You're not going to die, you know."

"That's what you think," I muttered. I pulled on the bras, one after another. None of them fit. They were all too big. Earthworm sized tears snaked down my face until my eyes swelled shut and my nose turned red.

"What are you doing in there?" asked Mom. She unceremoniously yanked back the curtain. "Oh good grief, you can't try on a bra over your undershirt."

Unable to speak through the mucous and humiliation, I gave the bras back to my mother.

"They don't fit. I don't want you in here. I want to go home."

Mom closed the curtain and I put my sweater back on. When I came out, she was holding a package. "Let's get some tea."

We went to the tearoom with red velvet wallpaper on the store's fourth floor. Women sat in small groups drinking tea and eating cakes from the trolley pushed by a woman with an enormous bosom.

"I bet you want me to look like that. I'm never going to look like that."

"Well I should hope not," said my mother. "Look around you. Women come in all shapes and sizes."

While the women were wearing the same style of clothes as my mother, I saw myself surrounded by a feast of breasts. From smoothly iced cupcakes decorated with tiny sprinkles to scones heavy with cream and studded with prominent raisins, the array was dazzling and mesmerizing.

"You know better than to stare."

"I can't do anything right," I said blubbering again. In this respectable room, my tears, slitty eyes and red nose were politely ignored. Properly raised Brits burrow emotion into our conversational word choice. The superlatives, "quite marvelous", "absolutely fabulous", and the ever-present "brilliant, absolutely brilliant", said with a straight face were accepted expressions of mild to acute emotional exuberance in Britain. Crying was not an accepted expression.

"Act like a young lady." And with that, my mother opened her purse to give me an intricately embroidered lace-edged handkerchief.

When I had dabbed up as much of the tears and other body fluids as possible, I inspected the tearoom. The combined smells of tannin, treacle, talc and lipstick hung in the room. I knew these women and their smells. My mother slid me a sideways look, straightened my sweater, and then she did something completely out of character. With an unexpected twinkle in her eyes, my mother told me how she almost married a comedian from the West End of London. "His name was Edward. He was very handsome."

"Really? Was he on the telly?"

"Yes. He had his own show."

"Ooooh. What's his last name?" I was 'all ears' never having heard this story from my mother.

"His name was Edward Bsor... " She tried again.

"Edward ... Bsgrrwe ... " Mother choked on her cake trying to pronounce his last name. "Welsh. He was Welsh. Lots of consonants." Crumbs scattered across her bosom.

I stuck my nose in the air and enunciated with my best upper class tone. "You were affianced to ... Edward Bsorrrgh ... Edwa ... "

"Eddie ... " She wiped the crumbs off her sweater.

"Eddie Funny Last Name."

"I was going to be Mrs. Eddie Funny Last Name," and my mother tittered.

"I would have been their daughter, Trudi Funny Last Name," and I snickered.

"We should put our mind to it. Let me try again. I would have been – Mildred ... Bsorrngwrrrerrth." Mother almost strangled on the consonants and cake.

We tried to pronounce the name. We really truly tried. Neither of us could pronounce the name.

"You would have been Mildred What's-Her-Name."

"And you would have been Trudi What's-Her-Name."

We giggled like schoolgirls. Tea shot out of my nose. Mother continued to choke on cake, finally spitting it into her napkin. We understood the impossibility of marrying a man with an unpronounceable last name. Our laughter became louder, turning heads in the tearoom. We couldn't stop. When the tea trolley woman asked if we were done, my proper mother snorted. Sanctioning eyes followed us. She gave me back my Mogen David and kissed me on the top of my head – probably the least snotty part of my body. In that moment, I loved my mother.

Her laughter made me realize there will always be things shared only with other women and unknowable to men. She had initiated me into womanhood. The Marks & Spencer bras may not have fit but in this memory my mother and I do.

Later, I found out my mother had bought a bra. After I went to bed, she undid all the machine-sewn seams and remade the bra with her tiny uneven stitches. She had another surprise for me – she bought my first adolescent outfit. It was a yellow knit top, hot pants, and striped tights. The newly fashioned bra added just the right curve to the top's clingy fabric.

The next day, dressed in my new clothes and bra, I proudly displayed my transformed body to the women of my family. They stood and applauded.

"Bloody fantastic," said my sister.

"You'll turn heads and break hearts in that get up," cried Granny.

"Brilliant, absolutely brilliant," said my cousin.

Mom looked on smiling. I hugged her and joined the circle of women. My crabby teenage heart was overwhelmed with my mother's gifts of femininity, laughter, and complicity. That bra would fit my body for six months and always fit in my heart, unlike the more difficult fit with my mother.

    I often wonder if Princess Anne wore that same yellow bra and if the Queen bought it for her.

First Crop

Females and males have breasts. Both sexes have nipples and areolas.

In females, as early as 8 and usually by 9 or 10, breast buds begin to rise from the girl's flat chest. The buds are about the size of a quarter. They contain fat and gland tissue that will develop over the next three to five years into what we label breasts. The buds may grow at uneven rates and signal the beginning of puberty with the arrival of a girl's period on average around two years later.

Boys are reaching puberty six months to two years earlier (at ages nine or ten) than the average age of eleven from a decade ago. Forty percent of boys develop significant breasts due to the hormonal changes of puberty. In 90% of these boys, the breasts will disappear within three years or less. Many young boys wonder if there is something wrong with them and feel acute shame.

In both sexes, breasts may tingle and be tender. Hair may grow around the areolas and nipples. Some people get stretch marks from the growth of their breasts. Development of breast tissue usually develops at the same time as the arrival of hair under the arms and in the pubic area. These are normal signs of puberty in girls and boys.

References:

Bellock, Pam. "Boys Now Enter Puberty Younger, Study Suggests, but It's Unclear Why." *The New York Times* 20 Oct. 2012: n. pag. Print.

CYWH staff, Boston's Children's Hospital. "Normal Breast Development." *Center for Young Women's Health: Health Information for Teen Girls around the World*. Boston's Children Hospital, 8 July 2010. Web. 4 Jan. 2013. <http://www.youngwomenshealth.org/breast_health_normal.html>.

CYWH staff, Boston's Children's Hospital. "Breast Health." *Center for Young Women's Health: Health Information for Teen Girls around the World*. Boston's Children Hospital, 29 Aug. 2013. Web. 27 Oct. 2013. <http://www.youngwomenshealth.org/breast_health.html>.

Herman-Giddens, Marcia E., Jennifer Steffes, Donna Harris, Eric Slora, Michael Hussey, Steven A. Dowshen, Richard Wasserman, Janet R. Serwint, and Lynn Smitherman. "Secondary Sexual Characteristics in Boys: Data from the Pediatric Research in Office Settings Network." *Pediatrics* 2011 (2012): 3291. *Pediatrics.aappublications.org*. Web. 1 Jan. 2013.

Klass, Perri. "Needed: More Attention to Boys' Development." *The New York Times* 7 Jan. 2013: Health. Print.

Marshall, W A., and J. M. Tanner. "Variations in Patterns of Pubertal Changes in Girls." *Archives of Disease in Childhood* 44.235 (1969): 291-303. Web. 4 Jan. 2013.

Marshall, W A., and J. M. Tanner. "Variations in the Pattern of Pubertal Changes in Boys." *Archives of Disease in Childhood* 45.239 (1970): 13-23. Web. 4 Jan. 2013.

"Tanner Scale." *Wikipedia: The Free Encyclopedia*. Wikimedia Foundation, Inc., 2013. Web. 7 Nov. 2012. <http://en.wikipedia.org/wiki/Tanner_scale>.

"Training Bra." *Wikipedia*. 2012. *Wikimedia Foundation, Inc.*. Web. 4 Jan. 2013. <http://en.wikipedia.org/wiki/Training_bra>.

Activity 1

With a friend or in a journal, talk or write about when you first noticed you had breasts.

> How old were you?
>
> What were you doing when you noticed?
>
> Who did you tell?
>
> Was the information celebrated, ignored, or a source of shame?
>
> What will/did you tell your daughter or son?

Activity 2

Set a timer for three minutes.

Write down the alternative and slang names you know for the word BREAST. Each word should go on a different note card.

Arrange the note cards into three categories

> ACCEPTABLE to say in front of a preteen or teenage girl or boy
>
> UNACCEPTABLE to say in front of a preteen or teenage girl or boy
>
> UNSURE if I should say in front of a preteen or teenage girl or body

With a friend or group of friends, discuss what characteristics distinguish the categories?

Resources:

CYWH staff, Boston's Children's Hospital. "Normal Breast Development." *Center for Young Women's Health: Health Information for Teen Girls around the World.* Boston's Children Hospital, 8 July 2010. Web. 4 Jan. 2013. <http://www.youngwomenshealth.org/breast_health_normal.html>.

CYWH staff, Boston's Children's Hospital. "Breast Health." *Center for Young Women's Health: Health Information for Teen Girls around the World.* Boston's Children Hospital, 29 Aug. 2013. Web. 27 Oct. 2013. <http://www.youngwomenshealth.org/breast_health.html>.

Dharam Kaur, Sat. "Breast Health Tips for Teens: Early Intervention Strategies in Preventing Breast Cancer." *The Healthy Breast Program.* MammAlive.net, 2013. Web. 4 Jan. 2013. <http://www.mammalive.net/sites/mammalive.net/files/Breast%20Health%20Tips%20for%20Teens.pdf>.

www.gynecomastia.com (information about male breast formation)

www.mammalive.com (breast health tips for teens with a focus on cancer prevention)

Weiss, M C., and I. Friedman. *Take Care of Your Girls*. New York, NY: Three Rivers Press, 2008. Print.

www.youngwomenshealth.org (health information for teen girls around the world)

A Prehistoric Bug

Lenny knew of Lizzie's reputation but wanted to take her on a proper date anyway. He wondered what other people would think of him when word got out. Would he be a stud, gaining status? Would the girls with good reputations still want to go out with him? Would he be contaminated? He didn't know who to talk to about this.

But Lizzie had always been kind to him and he appreciated that. She said hello to him in the halls and made him laugh during French.

"Hey your paper's on the floor," she said.

"Merci, beaucoup," he said.

"Don't let old lady Sanderson catch you without your homework," and she had winked at him, taking folders from her very neat locker before slipping through the packed hall. He watched her walk through the school hallway envying every person she bumped into.

One day, Lizzie smiled at him as he walked by with his friends. He looked down for a step then pretend-punched his friend in the arm. Lizzie stopped in front of him.

"Hi," Lizzie said.

"Uh, hi," he said and moved on.

"Do you know her?" The friend had asked.

Lenny tripped over his own High-tops.

"School slut. Don't know her," the friend said.

Lenny looked back at her as he kept pace with his friends. Lizzie bit her lip and hugged her book bag closer to her body.

The next time he saw her was at the Sadie Hawkins Dance. Last dance before their senior prom. When his date went to the rest room, Lenny made his way to Lizzie watching the crowd from the bleachers.

"Hi," he said.

"Hello," she said.

"I meant to say hi the other day … "

"Yeah, I heard your friend."

During French class the next week, Lizzie pinged a paper football at his head. He swore at her, "Zut alors." They giggled. He thought she must have forgiven him.

The teacher called them to the front of the class to act out the silly little dialogue of the week. In this scripted conversational, Lizzie had to ask Lenny where he kept his sausages, "Ou est les saucises?" She tried four times. He laughed. She laughed with him. Soon the whole class was laughing. Love's Baby Soft perfume floated up to him. "I'll take the F," she said to the teacher. Lenny admired her guts.

As the school year passed, Lizzie started to take on this allure. She slid through classes in her tight jeans and goofy tee shirts. Moving through squares of sunlight and sudden shadows, Lenny saw her body as a dancing mosaic of breasts and ass. Sitting in class, she was framed in soft light, like the sun decided to laugh with her. Little sparkles caught in her brown hair, settled on her shoulders and glowed on her chest. She was too golden to look at - too lovely to look away from.

It was after French class one Spring Tuesday, Lenny seriously considered asking Lizzie out. He talked with his best friend. "What do you think would happen if I asked Lizzie out?"

"You'd get a disease," his friend said.

"You think?"

"Yeah, I think. She's gone out with a lot of guys. Cute though. Great boobs. Could see why you'd want some of that."

"You're probably right," Lenny said. But the tantalizing thought of taking Lizzie out, sitting with the golden sparkles and sweet clean smell of her rolled around in his brain.

At the next French class, Lizzie leaned over him, correcting his homework. Little pools of light danced off her breasts. When he could look down her tee shirt, he was fascinated by the white tan lines criss-crossing tawny skin. He may have asked in French, probably English.

"Do you wanna go to the Elton John concert Saturday?"

"Avec vous?"

His brain jammed with images and thoughts and verb conjugations. He saw the edge of a lacy bra and knew he wanted to touch her. Lenny shifted in his seat. He was fidgeting with impatience.

She looked up at him, cocked her head to one side, said, Yes." With a knowing smile, she moved in her seat obstructing his view.

"What time are you going to pick me up?"

"What time does the concert begin?"

"Begins at eight."

"Pick me up at seven."

"When do you have to be home?"

"My curfew's midnight."

"Do you think you could stay out later? Traffic. You know."

Lenny tried to pull his gaze from her breasts. He wanted to take her out for the right reasons.

"I'll ask," she said frowning and turned back to her notes.

Lenny didn't tell anyone he was taking Lizzie out. The night of the concert, he was nervous. The car was full of gas, every surface glossy clean. He had stripped the pine tree air freshener from the rearview mirror wanting the full Lizzie experience, bioluminescence and pheromones, two newly learned words from biology class. He carefully shaved and borrowed a twenty from his Dad. Mom looked at him curiously like she knew he was going to do something … bad.

"She must be quite a girl, Lenny."

"I think she is, Mom."

"They're all good at that age," said his Dad from the den's darkness. "Go have fun but be careful."

"Dad," he groaned appalled that his thoughts were so apparent.

Lenny's mom reached out to him before he left. "Be a good guy," she said, passing him another twenty dollars. "Take her out for a burger afterwards."

Lizzie met him at her door wearing jeans and one of those halter-tops with ties at the neck and back. He kept staring at the vee where the fabric was tight.

"Back up a little," she said. He took a step backwards—eyes still focused on her halter and stumbled.

"Be careful," she said, echoing his father's words.

At the concert, his fingers moved continuously, practicing untying knots. He was deaf to the music. She talked to him and he had a hard time understanding her words.

Later, they sat on his car with cups of Coca Cola spiked with Southern Comfort. She threw an ice chip at him and he pretended to pour his drink over her head.

"I thought you didn't like me," she said.

"I've always liked you," he said wetting his fingers with the booze. She watched intently. He licked the bourbon from his fingers. He put two fingers over the bottle and turned it upside down. Her eyes were wide and luminous in the velvet night as he placed his fingers to her lips. Her cat-like tongue curled and licked the booze into her mouth. His lips followed, tasting Southern Comfort and Coca Cola with a sunlight kick. Next he put bourbon-covered fingers at the base of her throat and slowly ran them down vulnerable skin into the vee. She shuddered and pulled away.

"Don't."

"Why not?"

"I don't do that."

"I'm not asking you to do anything."

"Yes, you are," she said getting into the car.

They drove home in congealed silence. Lizzie looked out the window.

"I didn't mean to upset you," Lenny said, just as upset as she. She turned back to him, pupils dilated with bourbon tears.

He reached out to touch the tiniest edge of her jeans. She turned away, arms crossed against her chest.

"You think I'm a slut. I know what they say about me."

"What?" he stammered.

"They say I'm easy just because I have big breasts. It's been this way since junior high. That's why you asked me out isn't it?"

"No, course not. I, I wanted to go to the concert with someone fun."

"Promise. Promise that's true."

He was silent. "It's mostly true," he said. She started to cry.

"You don't know me, but I know you," she said. It was the biggest accusation of his life.

At her house, Lenny walked Lizzie to the door just as a palmetto bug flew at them. Lenny swatted at the flying roach. Its brown wings fluttered as it tried to alight. Lizzie stood still and the filthy prehistoric insect landed right on the spot he had coveted, traced and defiled.

Lizzie looked directly at Lenny. The roach started to crawl down the valley between Lizzie's breasts. Under the radiant skin, her jaw hardened. She undid the halter's knot at the back. Reaching under the top, she flicked away the bug between her breasts. Lenny caught a flash of full breasts.

"There. At least you can say you saw them," Lizzie said, retying her halter.

Lenny's mouth fell open. Her breasts had been perfect. Beyond his dreams. So much better than his father's Playboy fantasies.

"Close your mouth. The bug might come back."

Lenny started to stammer. Lizzie stepped into her house and closed the screen door between them.

"But I want to see you again?"

The insect buzzed around Lenny's head before landing

on the screen. The large brown bug was silent. Smooth armored back to him. A guardian.

Lizzie wasn't finished.

"I thought you were different. You liked me for me. I wouldn't have gone out with you if I thought you were just like the other boys."

Lizzie latched the screen door, turned away and slammed the front door shut. Lenny was left standing on the porch alone.

Lenny drove home carefully, more from the shame than the bourbon. His mother's twenty taunted him. The closer he got to home, the louder it became until it was screaming out, "What made you think you could do that? What are you going to do now? What if she talks to her friends?"

Quietly he opened the door and stepped sneakily to the stairs. "How'd it go?" called his father from the TV lit den. His mom stopped running water in the kitchen to listen. Lenny grunted and ran up to his room. He heard his father hoist himself out of the recliner saying, "Guess it didn't go so well."

Lenny told his Dad an edited version of the night with the usual teenage bravado. "She was so pretty, Dad. We had fun at the concert. I took her to a place to … you know … talk. Had to fight off this enormous bug at her house. It started to go down her halter … " Lenny looked away.

"What's the problem then?" His Dad leered.

"The bug got more than I did." Lenny knew he had failed at masculine swagger in his Dad's evaluation. He looked up to see his still young mother standing in the doorway, arms crossed over her breasts.

She looked between the two males. Biting her top lip, she rubbed her wedding ring side to side.

"Here," said Lenny handing back the twenty to his mother. "We didn't get the burgers."

Lenny's mother took the twenty by the very edge of the bill.

"Were you a good guy?"

"Good as guys get," said his Dad.

A Prehistoric Bug

August 26, 2012 was designated as International Go Topless Day. It was the fifth annual event that took part in 30 cities throughout the US from Asheville, NC to New York City. Small numbers of women went topless or covered their nipples with red tape. Men were encouraged to wear bikini tops in support. A few men participated in the activity. While men can go topless without legal or societal sanctions, when working in the yard, working out in gyms, taking class in yoga studios or even walking down the street, in nineteen US states, it is illegal or unclear about the legality of showing the female breast in public.

During events for International Go Topless Day in 2012, more men than women came to watch the parades. The men harassed the women, calling them 'slut' and 'whore', chasing them down the street and grabbing at their breasts. Some women, the topless protestors and the on-lookers, ran from the parade sites to avoid the bullying, misogyny, and assault.

A new term was developed for this behavior called "slut bashing." It is a form of bullying and sexual harassment using insults (at the least) to shame, degrade, and dehumanize females of all ages based on actual or perceived sexual behavior.

- 70% of female middle school and high school students experience "slut bashing" or other forms of sexual harassment.

- The Urban Dictionary (www.urbandictionary.com) defines "Slut" as a derogatory term for a sexually promiscuous female or "a female with the morals of a male."

The rigid division of girls based on perceived and actual sexual activities categorizes girls into good girls and bad girls, the Madonna/Whore Complex, or the Ho vs. Housewives split. Research shows this polarization leads to decreased self-esteem, increased promiscuity, increased sexual risk taking, depression, self-harm activities, and in two reported cases from Florida and Massachusetts, suicide. Girls whose bodies develop before their classmates or are more developed (for example, their breasts are bigger than their peers) are more often labeled as sluts and at risk for slut bashing/sexually harassing behavior. This occurs at an age when girls and boys are developing a sexual identity, learning how to ask for what they need and want sexually, and take charge of their own safety from STDs and unwanted pregnancies.

This sexual double standard and the resultant name calling psychologically damages young people and hinders necessary teenage developmental tasks.

References:

Palmer, Brian. "When Did Bare Breasts Become Taboo? Topless Kate Middleton Photos Would Have Been Socially Acceptable in Some Eras." *Explainer: Answers to Your Questions About the News*. Slate.com, 19 Sept. 2012. Web. 1 Jan. 2013. <http://www.slate.com/articles/news_and_politics/explainer/2012/09/kate_middleton_topless_photos_when_did_bare_breasts_become_taboo_.html>.

Stamoulis, Kathryn. "The New Teen Age." *Slut Bashing*. Psychology Today, 10 June 2010. Web. 4 Jan. 2013. <http://www.psychologytoday.com/blog/the-new-teen-age/201006/slut-bashing>.

Tannenbaum, Leora. *Slut! Growing Up Female with A Bad Reputation*. New York, NY: HarperCollins, 2000. Print.

Tannenbaum, Leora. "Two So-Called Sluts, Two Deaths, Only One Uproar." *The Huffington Post* 13 Apr. 2010: Healthy Living. Web. 4 Jan. 2013. <http://www.huffingtonpost.com/leora-tanenbaum/two-so-called-sluts-two-d_b_533425.html>.

Valenti, Jessica. *The Purity Myth: How America's Obsession with Virginity is Hurting Young Women*. Berkeley, CA: Seal Press, 2009. Print.

Activity 1

Three people are to take the roles of Lenny, Lenny's father, and Lenny's mother.

Finish the scene – Lenny is talking to his father and his mother is watching.

What would Lenny's mother say to Lenny?

What would Lenny's father say to his wife, Lenny's mother?

What would the father and mother's interaction be teaching Lenny about adult relationships and the expectations of the different genders?

Activity 2

Two people are to take the roles of Lizzie and Lizzie's mother.

Have Lizzie describe what happened.

What could Lizzie's mother say that would comfort Lizzie?

What would this situation teach Lizzie about adult relationships and the expectations of the different genders?

As a team, brainstorm what would be helpful to teach adolescents about body development. Formulate some ideas of what would be helpful to teach adolescents about sexuality during the school years and beyond.

Activity 3

Play the Telephone/Gossip Game.

With people seated in a circle, have one person (the Origin) whisper a statement into the ear of the person on their right. (The left ear has a more difficult time interpreting speech correctly.)

Possible statements to start with are:

Girls with big breasts are –

Good girls don't –

Bad girls will –

Good guys don't –

Bad guys do –

Guys who go out with girls with large breasts are –

Guys who go out with bad girls are –

Then that person whispers into her/his neighbor's left ear (the person on their right side) what she or he heard. Whispering from one person to the next continues around the circle until it comes back to the Origin/first person who says aloud the original and the "gossiped" statement. Write down the two statements. After as many rounds as you would like, discuss:

If you were talking about your sister/daughter/mother, would these statements be embarrassing or hurtful?

If you were talking about your brother/son/father, would these statements be embarrassing or hurtful?

What would it feel like to have this said about you?

How would it impact your behavior?

What values and/or stereotypes are you promoting or condoning?

When is it okay to repeat a story when you know that it has probably been changed or will be changed in the process of telling it?

Activity 4

Gather a group of people and give each person five slips of paper and a black pen.

Each person writes a different statement they have said or heard about another person on a different slip of paper.

Participants are reminded to omit names of the person they are writing about or to use fake names.

The slips of paper are collected in a bowl to ensure some privacy.

A person reads each slip and the group classifies each statement as:

    Bullying

    Sexual harassment

    Gossip

    Harmless

The group can develop definitions of the classifications and outline the characteristics of each classification.

Resources:

www.goodmenproject.com (a website explicitly exploring masculinity in the 21st century)

www.gotopless.org

www.kidshealth.org (sections for parents, kids, and teenagers)

www.stopbullying.gov (website with sections for LGBT youth and information on policies and laws)

www.stopsexualbullying.com

www.teenlineonline.org (chat line for teens talking with other teens)

Visual Coffee Breaks

Perplexed, she watched him go to lick his hearing aid. "Your tits are interlopers. They intrude on my day. I'm sitting at my desk trying to get work done. Nine to six. Like before I ever saw your tits and then an image of them seizes my mind."

"Maybe it needs a new battery," she said. He focused on the small mechanical knob in his hand. Shaking his head, he put it down and started tightening his belt.

"I can't shake it. I can't get my work done. It takes twenty to thirty minutes to get back into my professional mindset."

She looked up at him from the bed, mildly amused as his hands fluttered in frustration. "Think of them as a visual coffee break," she said stretching, arms extended overhead, back arched.

"Stop that. I tell you, they intrude. I say to myself, I'll think of them at night, between six and ten thirty but they keep interrupting my workday. I'm so far behind." He stared long and hard. Finally getting the metal prong in his belt, he maneuvered the hearing aid in his ear. "Twenty to thirty minutes."

"Kind of long for a coffee break," she said. His hearing aid whined.

"They're like Pamela Anderson's."

"But they're real. Look they sag. My tits aren't anywhere near as big. Didn't she die?"

"No that was Anna Nicole Smith."

"So now you're keeping track of tits and their owners."

"Only the really beautiful ones. Do you know how beautiful you are?"

"If they are so discombobulating then maybe you should sleep with someone who is less beautiful," she said from the sheets.

"What?" he said fiddling with the hearing aide. He stepped to the bed reaching for the objects of his obsession. "I want your tits. I promise to take good care of them."

"You can't have them but you can have visitation rights." She slid onto her stomach creating a tantalizing crevice for his viewing.

"There are words for women like you."

"Fun. Honest. Sharing."

"Not exactly." He stroked. "My property. Maybe I should mark them so there's no confusion."

"You don't trust me?"

"Hmmm."

"Do you want a Sharpie?" she said rolling onto her side to present him with yet another view.

"Your glorious tits were the first thing I noticed about you during that fated lunch."

"I was wearing a dress," and she covered her tits.

"Yes but there they were. Distracting me. I couldn't eat."

"I wondered if you were having problems hearing me. You did eat a lot of biscuits, slathered with butter, dripping with honey."

"You ate the ham. All of the ham."

"Yeah, I like pig." They both laughed. "How do you sublimate and stay so slim?" Her hands played peek-a-boo.

"I only sublimate about your tits," and he bent down to kiss them.

"Is this why most men gain twenty to thirty pounds when they date me?"

"Wouldn't be surprised. One pound for every minute on a coffee break."

Visual Coffee Breaks

In mammals, breasts grow for feeding babies and then deflate when the babies are weaned. Only human females have enlarged breasts full time. And men pay attention to women's breasts. Research studies have shown that after looking at pictures of women's curves, men will perform poorly on tests of cognitive skills.

- Memory decreases.
- Problem solving ability decreases.
- Brain centers associated with the rewards of alcohol and drugs are activated.

Men are rewarded for their visual evaluation and preoccupation with female curves. Hugh Hefner knows this and has the bank account to prove it. Women know this. In times of economic recession, in theory, women show more cleavage to compete for limited mating resources and to guard their mates from other women.

Women aspire to look like Barbie dolls. In the US, girls are given their first Barbie doll around the age of three and play with them until the onset of puberty, about age twelve. Yale and Duke Universities have calculated the statistics of a human Barbie. If Barbie were a real life woman, she would be over 7 feet tall, weigh 100 to 110 pounds, wear size 3 shoes and have bust/waist/hip measurements of 39/21/33 inches. These dimensions would place her in the dangerously anorexic category. She would be unable to walk upright. Yet this is one of the first models children are given of an adult woman.

Therefore, it is understandable that women overestimate the size of breasts that men prefer. While the average American woman is a 36D, up from 34B a generation ago, Barbie's 39 inch chest, 21 inch waist and 33 inch hips could be found in less than one in 100,000 of today's U.S. women.

Barbie is a figure well known to both sexes. Yoga instructors will call out "Barbie toes" to their students and most every woman in the class (and quite a few of the men) know the exact position of the feet with elongated ankle and flexed toes (the necessary foot position for wearing high heels).

	Barbie	**Average US Woman**
Height	7' 2"	5' 4"
Weight	100-110#	140-150#
Shoe Size	3	8
Chest/Bust	39"	35.9" (36C)
Waist	21"	34-35"
Hips	33"	43-46"

When an average US woman compares herself with this first image of a female body, it is no wonder that Barbie has been nicknamed the "plastic bane of body image."

References:

Black, Rosemary. "Looking at Curvy Women's Bodies Has the Same Effect on Men as Taking Drugs: Study." *NY Daily News* 24 Feb. 2010: Health. Web. 4 Jan. 2013. <http://www.nydailynews.com/life-style/health/curvy-women-bodies-effect-men-drugs-study-article-1.195112>.

Duenwald, Mary. "Body and Image: One Size Definitely Does Not Fit All." *The New York Times* [New York] 22 June 2003: Health. Web. 4 Jan. 2013. <http://www.nytimes.com/2003/06/22/health/body-and-image-one-size-definitely-does-not-fit-all.html?pagewanted=all&src=pm>.

Kemp, Charlotte. "Why Can't Men See Past Our Breasts?" *Mail Online* [United Kingdom] 21 Mar. 2012: Femail. Web. 4 Jan. 2013. <http://www.dailymail.co.uk/femail/article-2118403/As-Susanna-Reid-bemoans-public-fixation-breasts-long-suffering-DD-cup-wearer-sympathises.html>.

Maine, Margo. *Body Wars*. Carlsbad, CA: Gurze Books, 2000. Print.

Platek, S M., and D. Singh. "Optimal Waist-to-Hip Ratios in Women Activate Neural Reward Centers in Men." *PLoSONE* 5.2 (2010): n. pag. Web. 4 Jan. 2013. <http://www.plosone.org/article/info:doi/10.1371/journal.pone.0009042>.

Slaven, Galia. "The Scary Reality of a Real-Life Barbie Doll." *Huff Post College*. The Huffington Post, 8 Apr. 2011. Web. 4 Jan. 2013. <http://www.huffingtonpost.com/galia-slayen/the-scary-reality-of-a-re_b_845239.html>.

Williams, Florence. "Breast Case Scenarios." *Oprah* May 2012: 138-140. Print.

Zernicke, Kate. "Sizing Up America: Signs of Expansion From Head to Toe." *The New York Times* 1 Mar. 2004: n. pag. Web. 21 Nov. 2012.

Activity 1

With another person, describe your breasts in detail and aloud. Your partner will write down your individual words on sticky notes. State the color, shape, size, skin texture, and anything else you have noticed. Pay attention to what you like and dislike.

What words did you stumble over?

What words were easy to say?

Arrange the notes from most comfortable to least comfortable to say aloud. Read them aloud again.

Explain to your activity partner where your descriptions come from – family, music, culture, media, friends, lovers, doctors and medical practitioners are some places we receive information about our breasts.

Change roles and repeat the exercise.

Activity 2

Using the words on the notes, write something about your breasts. You could:

1) Write a letter from your Older Self (from yourself in your 50s, 60s or 70s) to your breasts stating what you appreciate about them.

Read it aloud in front of a mirror.

2) Arrange some of the words on the note cards created in Activity 1 in a haiku (form of Japanese poem).

The first line will have 5 syllables.

The second line will have 7 syllables.

The third line will have 5 syllables.

Here are two examples from October Haikus in honor of breast awareness on the Collegiate Sports Nation website (CSNBBS):

> Boobs Titties Knockers
> Fun bags hooters cans udders
> So much fun to touch

> Or

> Boobies boobies boobs
> Boobies boobies boobies boobs
> Boobs boobies boobies

Read your haiku aloud. Say as a mantra (breath/sound meditation) 20 times. How do the words and your relationship to the words change after 20 readings?

Activity 3

Put the females on one side of the room and the males on the other side.

Males write down on a slip of paper the size breasts they think women prefer on themselves.

Females write down on a slip of paper the size breasts they think men prefer.

Compare the information from the two groups.

> Were the two groups close?

Why did you choose that particular size?

What if you are a different size?

What if you like a different size?

What have you learned about yourself, your gender group, and the other gender group?

Resources:

Braddock, Carolyn J. *Body Voices*. Berkeley, CA: PageMill Press, 1995. Print.

Joannides, Paul, and Daerick Gross, Sr. *The Guide to Getting It On*. 6th ed. Oregon: Goofy Foot Press, 2011. Print.

www.mensworx.com (website explaining heterosexual men's fascination with female breasts)

Unforced Errors

The best ball players at the club were indulging in their post-match ritual lubricated with at least two gin and tonics.

"She can return a ball," the blond man said.

"Maybe forehand but her backhand needs work," said the other man unsticking his legs. Both men were still slick with game sweat and the movement created the sound of a ball sliding down a wet court.

"Good ground strokes."

"Yep, and a mean slice on a ball if she needs to," and they both shifted forward to watch a low volley. The ball whacked the racquet's sweet spot with a thick twang.

"What color do you think her nipples are?"

"Can't tell. Damn those sports bras they wear now."

"Take a guess," he said leaning back.

"My guess would be brown. She's got the brown hair and dark tan of a woman who would be … brown." He looked away. The brown-haired woman returned the ball deep into the corner of her opponent's court.

"I think she's had a couple of kids. Too much baggage for me. Pink or no pink."

"Well she kept her shape. What about her opponent?"

"The blonde? Do you really think she's a blonde?"

"Never been close enough to know if her sofa and curtains match. You?"

"Nah. I want to marry a woman with pink nipples. No kids. Okay maybe one kid but the no pink nipples are a deal breaker." The steady rhythm of ball on racquet stopped.

"Wait a minute. She's bending over to pick up a ball."

"Which one, brown or possibly pink?"

"Someone needs to tell her not to flash the spectators or she'll get some unwelcome attention."

"Let her flash away." He stuck his hands in the damp pockets of his shorts.

"What you doing there, Mitch? Drying your hands?"

"Just making room for the boys," he smirked.

"Do you think they look up our shorts?"

"Of course not. They're women. Women don't do that."

"Why wouldn't they?"

"Well, they're women. They just want a nice house, some kids, and a good bang, when they want it."

"Do they know we're looking at them?"

Mitch snorted. "They know. They start planning in the cradle - from the cheerleaders to the little brainy college girls. Short skirts, tight sweaters, the ponytails that bob up and down. It's all advertising."

"Never thought of it that way. I feel like a babe in the woods," he said slapping his friend on the back. The blonde woman straightened up and stretched her racquet overhead.

"Feed me," said Mitch, mouthing a long suck. He took

off his shirt and puffed out his chest.

Women's laughter floated up from the courts. The two men straightened up and looked away. The ball resumed its course over the net with a rewarding thud.

"That was a bitchy look that woman gave us. Do you think they know we're talking about them?"

"Nah, probably talking about tampons or diapers or something." They sipped their drinks.

"Do you ever wonder if they talk about us?" Mitch choked on his drink and put on his shirt.

Unforced Errors

Breasts are found on the chests of males and females between the third and sixth or seventh ribs. The breast is a mammary gland capable of making colostrum and milk in a series of glands within fibrous connective tissue and covered with a layer of fat. A layer of connective tissue separates the breast from the pectoral muscles. The left breast is usually bigger than the right. Just below the center of the breast and protruding from the breast is the nipple. The nipple has several openings for colostrum and milk to flow through.

In the uterus, the fetus has two rows of nipples running down the right and left sides of the torso from the armpit to the groin. During the maturation process in the womb, most of the nipples disappear. At birth, most babies are born with two nipples and a few babies can produce milk. A third nipple is not uncommon. In adults, the third nipple cannot produce milk and usually looks like a mole.

Nipples have red and brown pigments called 'pheomelanin' (the red pigment) and 'brown eumelanin' giving it the pink to brown to very dark hue. Nipple shapes range from flat to round to cylindrical. The average human female nipple projects slightly more than 3/8 of an inch (10mm). A sensitive pigmented area called the areola surrounds a nipple. The areola's pigmentation can range from very pale, blending in with the skin of the breast, to very dark red or brown hued. The size of the areola can range from a small ring around the nipple to an area that covers half of a smaller breast. Montgomery glands on the areola are skin glands ranging in appearance from unnoticeable to prominent bumps. Montgomery Glands are thought to lubricate the nipple and areola. Usually, pregnancy makes the glands more pronounced. Some nipples have a few hairs around them.

In human females, areola and nipple color and size vary among individuals and over an individual's lifetime. Areola and nipple color and size do not correlate with breast size. In early puberty, areolas enlarge into 'buds' then flatten out in late puberty. Pregnancy and nursing can increase the nipple size and deepen pigmentation.

Like goosebumps, there can be many reasons for the contraction of the areola and the nipple. The areola can redden in hot weather due to increased circulation. When cold, irritated or stimulated, the muscular ability of the areola contracts the tissue and the nipple becomes erect, everts, gets hard or becomes an outie. Just because a woman has everted or hard nipples does not mean she is sexually excited. Just because a woman's nipples do not become everted or hard does not mean she is not sexually excited.

Some women have one or both nipples inverted. The inverted nipple points inward or appears to turns itself inside. It can look like a line was drawn through the nipple. This is not a cause for alarm. If a usually everted or outie nipple suddenly inverts, you should contact your medical provider.

Men have nipples. In the uterus, males and females begin with similar tissues and body parts including nipples. When a male embryo is six weeks old in the uterus, testosterone masculinizes the embryo prompting the growth of a penis and testicles but the vestigial nipples do not go away nor change much past this point. In certain situations, especially from the hormonal fluctuations of puberty or illness, males can develop noticeable breasts, produce milk and develop breast cancer.

References:

Feingold, David. "Pediatric Endocrinology." *Atlas of Pediatric Physical Diagnosis*. 2nd ed. Philadelphia, PA: W.B. Saunders, 1992. 9.16-19. Print.

"Female Intelligence Agency Examines: Normal Nipple Concerns and A Gallery." *Female Breasts: For Men or For Breastfeeding?* 007 Breasts, n.d. Web. 4 Jan. 2013. <http://www.007b.com/nipple_gallery.php>.

Gray, H, T. P. Pick, and R. Howden. *Gray's Anatomy*. Philadelphia, PA: Running Press Book Publishers, 1974. Print.

Kennard, Jerry. "Why Do Men Have Nipples: Why Have Male Nipples Not Disappeared?" *Men's Health*. About.com, 22 Mar. 2010. Web. 4 Jan. 2013. <http://menshealth.about.com/od/conditions/a/Nipples_Men.htm>.

Pinkola Estes, Clarissa. *Women Who Run With The Wolves*. New York, NY: Ballantine Books, 1992. Print.

Activity 1

For years, people have traveled to a mesa in New Mexico to watch "The Butterfly Dance." At the end of a long, hot, and tiring day trudging up the hill, an old woman comes out to touch everyone with her dance. The legend states she carries the "thunderworld in one breast" and the "underworld in the other" [Estes, M.P. (1992). Women Who Run With The Wolves. Ballantine Books: New York: NY. p. 211].

What do you carry in your breasts?

What would they say to you?

What would the right breast say to your left breast? Your left breast to your right?

Have your breasts ever surprised you?

Activity 2

Describe a beautiful breast. In detail. Aloud.

Size

Shape

Color of nipple and areola

Is this pornographic, erotic, artful, or medical? Name three individuals breasts' you find beautiful. Think about the people you know, celebrities, see in magazines, movies, and TV, etc.

What makes their breasts beautiful? Literally stand out?

Do these breasts belong to women, men, Caucasians, people of color and all the ethnicities you know or to a very specific group?

Marissa Pinkola Estes's wrote, "There cannot be one kind of breast, one kind of waist, one kind of skin," (Estes, p. 202).

Why would she say that?

Activity 3

Alone or with a partner, take out three sheets of paper. On each sheet, draw a large circle. (This activity is modified from an activity in Knopf and Seiler's book, <u>Inhibited Sexual Desire</u>, see Resource List.)

Label the first circle "Breast Activities I do now and enjoy"

Label the second circle "Breast Activities I don't do now but would like to try"

Label the third circle "Breast Activities I don't do now and don't want to try"

Fill in your circles with details of behaviors and activities. Be creative. Brainstorm. Be specific. Examples could include "buy a new bra," "rub oil into them," "pierce my nipples," "get a mammogram," "get fitted for a bra," and "have my partner suck my nipples."

First read them aloud to yourself.

Next share them by giving the sheets to your partner/friend

or by reading them to your partner/friend.

    Ask if your partner would share their list.
Listen with respect and care. Do not attack, criticize or shame yourself or the other person by labeling the items on the lists as 'disgusting," "weird," or "perverted."

    Ask for clarification when you don't understand.
Pay attention to the items in the second circle.

    What stops you from doing them?

    Who stops you from doing them?

    What would make it possible, even probable, you would be willing to try them?

The goal is to develop or increase your understanding of personal feelings, thoughts, and behaviors about breasts (and easing some of the anxiety around asking for what you want and need around breast play).

Resources:

www.imaginis.com/breast-health-non-cancerous/breast-anatomy-and-physiology (source of information about breast health and appearance)

Kennard, Jerry. "Why Do Men Have Nipples: Why Have Male Nipples Not Disappeared?" *Men's Health*. About.com, 22 Mar. 2010. Web. 4 Jan. 2013. <http://menshealth.about.com/od/conditions/a/Nipples_Men.htm>.

Knoft, Jennifer and Michael Seiler. *Inhibited Sexual Desire*. New York, NY: The Philip Lief Group, Inc. of Warner Books, 1990. Print.

www.mensworx.com (website from a heterosexual male viewpoint explaining men's fascination with women's breasts)

Pinkola Estes, Clarissa. *Women Who Run With The Wolves*. New York, NY: Ballantine Books, 1992. Print.

www.007b.com (website with basic information and a large gallery of breast/nipple pictures with an emphasis on the importance of breastfeeding)

No Lying

"Doesn't this just beat the band?" Ellie trudged to the bathroom holding a file folder against her chest. "Oh, my silk blouse. I can't believe it."

In the bathroom, she lifted her face to the mirror and studied an altered reflection. "I have the peachy glow," she groaned noting the dewy skin with its hormonal flush over the nose and cheeks. Squaring her shoulders so her ribcage pushed against the newly tight band of her bra, she stared at the face and neck in the mirror checking for the telltale brown mask. "Okay, my neck doesn't look any different."

Deliberately, she looked straight ahead. No premature peeking. "Maybe it's not what I think it is." Next, she studied the fit of her skirt in the mirror. "Nope, no change there." Then, shirt button by shirt button, she lowered the file, showing more and more of her reflection to herself. The silk shirt's fabric clung to twin wet spots on her chest, highlighting the breasts threatening to spill out of the bra's cups. "This can't be happening to me. Oh God, but it is." Ellie knew of no other explanation for the leaking breasts.

For a moment she covered her face with her hands then used them to prop herself against the sink. She looked full frontal into the mirror. The silk blouse was definitely going to draw attention when she left the bathroom. The file was sticky—her body having marked it with a thick yellow stain. Fighting the urge to giggle, maybe with embarrassment, maybe with joy, definitely with shock, Ellie wondered what to do next, what to think next.

"Not again." She drummed the fingers of her left hand against the countertop for several moments – mocked by the newly white band of skin on her finger. "Not now." Without awareness, she gnawed on the knuckles of her other hand.

"Guess I'll go home and change shirts." Ellie pressed her arms against her breasts, noticing the new round soreness. "They've grown." She hugged herself tighter. "I have cleavage, among other things." She noticed they had stopped leaking with the pressure from her arms and went into a stall to get some tissue paper. Her breasts felt too sensitive to tolerate the rough paper towels. After wetting the tissues in the sink, she returned to the stall, locked the door and took off her blouse. The lacy bra barely contained her breasts and didn't flatten out the distended nipples. "Well, this is useless." She took off the bra and looked down at her naked breasts, suddenly aware of the light threading of blue veins and newly ripe heft of her body. Reverently, she cleaned off the colostrum and patted her breasts dry.

While at first put off by the stain, the stickiness, and her breasts' new roundness, now Ellie was faced with the unmistakable message from her body. She weighed them in her hands. "Yep, they've grown. They leak. I can't avoid this. I'm pregnant." While her forehead scrunched, her lips smiled.

"Breasts don't lie."

No Lying

Breasts change with pregnancy. Breasts' fat glands and milk glands increase resulting in breast growth. Breasts can leak colostrum, the fluid made in your breasts before milk is made. Usually, colostrum is a clear and sweet tasting fluid. Colostrum can arrive as early as three or four weeks into a pregnancy but usually arrives midway through a pregnancy. Many women's breasts will start to leak between the 12th and 14th week of pregnancy and most commonly between the 26th and 30th week of pregnancy. By the third trimester, some women will start producing milk. Other women do not leak until after their baby is born. The time when breasts start to leak is not related to being able to produce milk nor breastfeed a baby. Leaking or spraying milk from the breasts can be in response to physical and emotional triggers.

Breastfeeding has always created moral, public health, economic, and political divisions. On one side of the division are the barriers against breastfeeding ranging from subtle processes of discouragement to the overt legal and societal barriers. Even with the American Academy of Pediatrics supporting breastfeeding as the healthy start for the first year of a child's life, less than half of American babies are breast fed for six months. The Academy states a baby/child should be weaned when the baby/child indicates they are ready. In 2004, a survey by the American Dietetic

Association found that only 43% of Americans believed women should be allowed to breastfeed in public. Images of women breastfeeding babies on the magazine *US Babytalk* have been found "gross" in roughly a quarter of the women polled in 2006.

As of May 2011, if a woman breastfeeds a child older than 12 months in the state of Tennessee, she can be arrested for public indecency. Target stores were the sites of organized "nurse-ins" after a woman was told she had to go to the fitting room to breastfeed her baby. In the virtual world, FaceBook has been quick to remove pictures of women breastfeeding their children under the "offensive content" or pornography rules from their Terms of Service agreement but took longer to deactivate an ad using a topless model for a dating service. Similar events have happened in other places from Applebee's to Wal-Mart to street festivals, from Kentucky to New York City to New Orleans, Louisiana.

On the other side of the division are various organizations and initiatives that support breastfeeding exemplified by La Leche League's pro-feeding stance to NYC Mayor Michael Bloomberg's hospital intervention. The international La Leche League is the major global organization lending support for breastfeeding. The League defines breastfeeding as natural, necessary, and satisfying for the mother and baby (see the La Leche League

Philosophy page at the llli.org website). They strongly encourage breastfeeding for nutrition and bonding of the baby with the mother. They want mother and baby together "early and often." The baby's father plays a large part in breastfeeding. His participation in the process bonds the couple's partnership while forming a "unique relationship with his baby." The father becomes a crucial nurturing figure in the child's development.

On a local level, New York City Mayor Bloomberg has proposed a breast-feeding initiative. Latch On NYC was his attempt to brand breast milk alternatives or baby formula as "dangerous medicine, only to be dispensed in case of emergency" (see the article by Rosin, 7/31/12). In hospitals, baby formula was to be kept locked away and only dispensed after a nurse had rigorously talked to the mother about the importance of breastfeeding her baby. Also, the reason why the baby was not breast-fed was noted in the woman's medical chart, a legal document that becomes part of the women's medical history, is attached to her Social Security Number, and can be subpoenaed.

American working women (and their female and male partners) have many reasons for not breast-feeding or using pumped breast milk. Reasons include lack of paid parental leave, inadequate break time to pump milk, lack of a supportive environment for pumping, and lack of storage areas for pumped breast milk.

The conflicting laws and organizations put women between a rock and a hard place. Breastfeeding is a legally enforced issue in some hospitals, not supported in the workplace, especially in companies with less than 50 employees, touted as the only nutritious method to feed a baby, forbidden in some areas, and infantilizes women when the decision to breastfeed is no longer is a matter of personal choice. Breastfeeding has become an issue of shame and criminal consequences not self-determination.

References:

www.aap.org/breastfeeding

"Breastfeeding In Public." *Wikipedia: The Free Encyclopedia*. Wikimedia Foundation, Inc., 2013. Web. 4 Jan. 2013. <http://en.wikipedia.org/wiki/Breastfeeding_in_public>.

The Labor of Love. "Leaking Breasts During the First, Second & Third Trimester." *TheLaborofLove*. Earth Magic Inc., n.d. Web. 4 Jan. 2013. <http://www.thelaboroflove.com/articles/leaking-breasts-during-the-first-second-third-trimester>.

www.llli.org (La Leche League International website)

Mollmann, Marianne. "Bloomberg's Breastfeeding Initiative: Let's Start with Paid Parental Leave." *The Huffington Post* 8 Aug. 2012: Parents. Web. 4 Dec. 2012. <http://www.huffingtonpost.com/marianne-mollmann/breastfeeding_b_1755188.html>.

NCSL.org. Breastfeeding Laws. (May 2011).

O'Connor, Mary. "Breastfeeding Benefits & Barriers: Breastfeeding Statistics in the United States." Breastfeedingbasics.org, 1998. Web. 16 Jan. 2013. <http://www.breastfeedingbasics.org/cgi-bin/deliver.cgi/content/Introduction/sta_us.html>.

Quart, Alissa. "The Milk Wars." *The New York Times* 14 July 2012: n. pag. Web. 4 Jan. 2013.

Rosin, Hanna. "Mayor Bloomberg Loves Breastfeeding More Than You Do." *What Women Really Think*. Slate, 31 July 2012. Web. 4 Jan. 2013. <http://www.slate.com/blogs/xx_factor/2012/07/31/new_york_mayor_bloomberg_s_new_breastfeeding_law_harmful_to_women.html>.

Sauer, Laura. "Bloomberg's Breastfeeding Initiative Bullies Mothers." *Yahoo! News*. Yahoo!, 3 Aug. 2012. Web. 4 Jan. 2013. <http://news.yahoo.com/bloombergs-breastfeeding-initiative-bullies-mothers-161300260.html>.

Activity 1

Write down all the comments, proverbs, religious and political statements you have heard about breastfeeding.

You can start with:

"It's the natural and right thing to do."

"Seeing your teeny, tiny, innocent baby latching on where only a lover has been before feels, well, a little creepy."

"Baby formula worked for generations of children."

"If you don't want to breastfeed, there is something wrong with your maternal instinct."

What do you feel about personally breastfeeding in public and seeing a woman breastfeeding in public?

Barbara Walters stated, "It made me very nervous" when a woman breast-fed her baby in the seat next to her on a plane.

What would you say to Barbara Walters?

What would you do if you were on a plane and needed to breastfeed or was seated next to someone breastfeeding?

Activity 2

Role-play a nurse talking to a new mother about why she should breastfeed her baby.

What would you include in the content of the speech?

What tone of speech (supportive, cajoling, punitive, etc.) would you use with the mother?

What would you do if the woman starts to cry or shout?

How would you respond to her decision?

What would you document in the woman's legal chart?

Activity 3

Develop a law for your state about breastfeeding.

Where can it happen – public, private, workplace, etc. – without legal consequences?

Does the women's nipple have to be covered when a baby/child is breastfed?

Is there an age limit on how old a baby/child can reach before it is considered illegal/indecent/inappropriate?

How will it be supported in the workplace? Are some workplaces exempt and why?

Should baby formula samples be included in the sample bags women get before leaving the hospital after giving birth?

Should Bloomberg's rules be enforced? And if so, how are the women to be punished?

Resources:

www.aap.org/breastfeeding (American Academy of Pediatrics: Dedicated to the Health of All Children website)

Bohling Smith, Pat, Karen Moore, and Liz Peters. "Implementing Baby-Friendly Practices: Strategies for Success." *The American Journal of Maternal/Child Nursing* 37.4 (2012): 228-233. Print.

La Leche League (international website is www.llli.org and in the US as www.lllusa.org)

McKeever, Joyce, and Rose St. Fleur. "Overcoming Barriers to Baby-Friendly Status: One Hospital's Experience." *Journal of Human Lactation* 28.3 (2012): 21-314. Print.

National Conference of State Legislatures has federal and state breastfeeding laws. NCSL.org (last updated May 2011).

www.thelaboroflove.com (a family of websites with blogs, research and answers to questions about starting a family)

A Wide Gap

"There are narrow and wide gaps on the axillary sternum."

"Excuse me," she said.

"Settle down. You moved too fast and the image bounced."

"Well shake the screen or something," she said staring hard into the computer.

"Looking at mammograms all day, I get excited to see a pair with a wide cleavage."

"And I have what kind of cleavage?" she said, searching her chest. The fast movements blurred the screen.

"You have a wide cleavage. Tilt the camera down so I can see again," he said lifting one eyebrow and one corner of his mouth.

"I don't think medical evaluation of breasts is why they invented Skype."

"Tilt the screen down. It'll be a tedious day. Full of anonymous breasts to evaluate."

"Feeling mammary overload? Weighed down in a sea of breasts? Adrift? Awash … "

He interrupted, "Are you making fun of my profession?"

"Of course not. Why would I make fun of a man complaining about evaluating breasts all day? And getting paid for it?"

"You're moving too fast again. I can't get a true read. Hold your breath and don't move."

"Very funny."

"Would you like a professional opinion on your breasts?" He leered into the camera. Up close his eyes looked crossed and his nose loomed enormous.

"So what happens if I have a narrow cleavage?"

"In a narrow cleavage, the medial portion of each breast is close to the other breast. The two breast tissues touch. Makes the mammogram more inclusive. Most films include the medial portions from narrow gaps. With your wide cleavage," and he drew out the word "wide" into a three syllable adjective, "your mammogram would be difficult to read."

"Maybe I should get gel inserts for my bra," she said hoisting up her breasts with a smile. "Then I'll fit in with your California double-d melons." She turned up one corner of her mouth and widened her eyes.

"Don't ever do that. Not around me. I do like those little Southern peaches." There was a Skype induced delay and his mouth turned down then up again. "We do ask the techs to tweak the nipple so we can have a good view," he said as his hands snaked out of camera range and his mouth turned up.

"Cleavage under my chin. Isn't that what men want?"

"Take your hands away. Your fruit are lovely the way they hang."

"I bet you say that to all the girls." She said smoothing her breasts.

"No, only the girls I want out of their bras. In fact, don't wear a bra around me ever."

"I'm at work. Shouldn't scare the coworkers."

"Stop bouncing on that yoga ball. I can't get a good image and it's distracting."

"Maybe you should take a breath," she dropped her voice.

"Lock the door," he said leaning in close to the camera.

"Are you sure you're a radiologist and not a plumber?"

"I'll plumb you," he said, twirling a make believe cigar and raising that eyebrow again.

"What did you say and why are your hands twitching?"

"Oh good grief. It's not that important."

"Are you wearing pants?" she asked.

"Want to see?" He started to rise out of his seat.

"No. No," covering her eyes with her hands. She peeked. He was still wearing the medical scrub top. His boys were pink from sitting in the fabric chair. She tapped an icon and the image filled her screen.

"Is that a narrow or wide cleavage?" she asked. He made little fishy kisses at the camera.

"You looked. I love how you peek through your long

fingers. Will you touch me with those fingers?"

"I don't think Skype will allow us to do that. But maybe if we got very close to the screen we could pretend."

"You like being virtually touched in the morning?"

"Hand check. Where are your hands? Spread 'em," she whispered into the screen.

"In your time zone, it must be near lunch. Back to your breasts. Yummy, yummy yummy, I've got love in my tummy. Take off your top."

"I told you, I can't do that at work. Maybe for your birthday."

"There are words for women like you."

"Fun, appropriate, afraid of having their breasts turn up on the Internet?" She watched his eyebrows reach new heights. "Be sure to put on your pants before going to work." She smirked on the screen.

"Take off your bra," he said smiling into the computer's camera.

A Wide Gap

Medical practitioners, their patients, and cosurvivors (family, friends, and caregivers of seriously ill patients) question the accuracy and safety of mammography. From the 1920s to the late 1960s, X-rays were used to evaluate problems of the chest and breast. In 1965 and 1966, Albert Salomon, named the inventor of breast radiology, along with Andre Willemin and Charles Gros founded the medical field of mammography. The first official mammogram was done in 1969.

Today, radiology technicians perform the mammograms. The films are read or interpreted by radiologists. A radiologist is expected to read around 53 mammograms per day and 260 in a week. Statisticians are examining the reliability and validity of mammograms and the accuracy of the radiologists reading them. With 40 years of data available, statisticians along with the medical community are beginning analyses of the gains of mammography against a growing list of problems including over-diagnosis, false positive and false negative results, and the effects of radiation exposure from mammography over a lifetime. A study completed in 2012 estimated breast cancer was over-diagnosed in 1.3 million patients in the last 30 years (or between 15% and 50% of cancers may be over-diagnosed depending on the study cited).

Mammography is the major process for viewing the

breasts of a woman and under some circumstances, the breasts of a man. A mammography study is a series of x-rays with multiple functions. Mammograms can:

- establish a baseline of what a woman's breasts look like before any suspicion of change or disease,
- screen women at high risk of developing breast changes,
- diagnose changes in the breasts/chest felt by patients and/or their medical practitioners (further examination methods may be needed),
- and provide early detection of recurrent or metastatic cancer.

Mammograms are a cheap, non-invasive, and portable test available to large populations through medical offices, hospitals, and traveling mammography vans. During mammography, each breast is x-rayed in different positions with the breast compressed as flat as possible between a firm x-ray film holder and a stiff rectangle of plastic. Each x-ray takes a few seconds and people report different levels of discomfort with the procedure. To some degree, women can minimize the pain of the procedure by scheduling their mammogram studies for one week after her menstrual period. Some women have compared compression to having their breasts "slammed in a refrigerator door."

Mammograms are prescribed for all women. A

baseline mammogram is usually taken between 35 and 40 for healthy women without risk factors. Beyond age 40, a woman in the US is expected to get a mammogram every year or every two years for the rest of her life. In other countries, mammograms are ordered every two to three years beyond age 40. The medical community has presented mammograms as an effective method to reduce the breast cancer mortality rates in women aged 39 to 49. Regular mammography screening has been found to equalize the mortality rates between White and Black women in the US. Regular mammography of women from 50 to 69 reduces the breast cancer mortality rate within the range of 10 to 25 percent depending on the study cited. In certain patients, mammograms can detect breast cancer before the woman, her partner, or a medical practitioner can feel a lump. Overall, breast cancer mortality rates have dropped 40% in the last 30 years.

Even so, medical practitioners are starting to evaluate the effectiveness of mammography for certain age groups and types of cancer with some scientists saying the benefits of mammography before 50 do not outweigh the risks. The medical community is beginning to worry about the harm of repeated radiation exposure from the x-rays. Statisticians are tracking long-term consequences of the radiation exposure and considering if they contribute to the rising breast cancer rates. Improvements in the mortality rates have been attributed to increased patient awareness and advances in treatment more than screening mammography.

Women can choose to do a breast self-exam to become aware of the appearance and feel of their breasts from the collarbones to the ribcage. She can check for changes throughout her life by knowing her breasts. Women have found lumps and dimpling in their breasts leading to evaluation and treatment of breast cancer and other breast illnesses. Easy and detailed directions for a breast self-exam are found on the American Cancer Society's website.

References:

Bleyer, A, and H. G. Welch. "Study: 1.3 Million Overdiagnosed Breast Cancers in 30 Years." *New England Journal of Medicine* 367 (2912): 1998-2005. Web. 22 Nov. 2012.

Carney, P A., T. A. Bogart, B. M. Geller, S. Haneuse, K. Kerlikowske, D. S. Buist, R. Smith, R. Rosenberg, B. C. Yankaskas, T. Onega, and D. L. Miglioretti. "Association between Time Spent Interpreting, Level of Confidence, and Accuracy of Screening Mammography." *American Journal of Roentgenology* 198.4 (2012): 970-978. *MedPub.gov*. Web. 16 Jan. 2013. <http://www.ncbi.nlm.nih.gov/pubmed/22451568>.

Fernandez, Elizabeth. "High Rate of False-Positives with Annual Mammogram." *UCSF: Advancing Health Worldwide*. Ucsf.edu, 17 Oct. 2011. Web. 16 Jan. 2013.

Friedenson, Bernard. "Is Mammography Indicated for Women with Defective BRCA Genes? Implications of Recent Scientific Advances for the Diagnosis, Treatment, and Prevention of Hereditary Breast Cancer." *Medscape Multispecialty*. Medscape, 9 Mar. 2000. Web. 2 Jan. 2013. <http://www.medscape.com/viewarticle/408048>.

Grabler, P, D. Dupuy, J. Rai, S. Bernstein, and D. Ansell. "Regular Screening Mammography before the Diagnosis of Breast Cancer Reduces Black: White Breast Cancer Differences and Modifies Negative Biological Prognostic Factors." *Breast Cancer Research Treatment* 135.1 (2012): 549-553. *National Center for Biotechnology Information*. Web. 26 Oct. 2013. <http://www.ncbi.nlm.nih.gov/pubmed/22886477>.

Magnus, M C., M. Ping, M. M. Shen, J. Bourgeois, and J. H. Magnus. "Effectiveness of Mammography Screening in Reducing Breast Cancer Mortality in Women Aged 39-49: A Meta-Analysis." *Journal of Womens Health* 20.6 (2011): 845-852. *National Center for Biotechnology Information*. Web. 2 Jan. 2013. <http://www.ncbi.nlm.nih.gov/pubmed/21413892>.

"Mammography." *Wikipedia: The Free Encyclopedia*. Wikimedia Foundation, Inc., 2013. Web. 26 Oct. 2013. <http://en.wikipedia.org/wiki/Mammography>.

Activity 1

Say the word "BREAST" aloud 15 times in front of a mirror. What is the difference between the first time you said it and the last the word?

Is there a change in the level of loudness by the end of the exercise?

Is there a change in the level of comfort by the end of the exercise?

Activity 2

Say the word "BREAST" aloud 15 times to a friend/partner. What is the difference between the first time you said it and the last time you said the word?

Is there a change in the level of loudness?

Is there a change in the level of comfort for the person talking?

Is there a change in the level of comfort for the person listening?

Activity 3

Collect images of breasts from magazines, postcards, and any place you find them. Don't edit. Tear them out. Notice if you want to leave some out or pretty them up.

Arrange them into a collage on a large piece of poster board, flipchart sheet, or piece of cardboard. The images that are important go in the center of picture. Less important images can be placed in the periphery or corners or outside edges of the picture.

> What's in the center and what's on the periphery?
>
> What personal values have you depicted in your collage?
>
> What's in the center and what's on the periphery?
>
> What societal values have you depicted in your collage?

Resources:

www.cancer.org/cancer/breastcancer/detailedguide/breast-cancer-detection (information on how to perform a breast self exam).

Mayo Clinic Staff. "Mammogram: How You Prepare." *Mayo Clinic: Health Information*. Mayo Foundation for Medical Education and Research, n.d. Web. 27 Nov. 2013. <http://www.mayoclinic.com/health/mammogram/MY00303/DSECTION=how-you-prepare>.

"Preparing for Your First Mammogram." *Kotex*. Kimberly-Clark Worldwide, Inc., 2013. Web. 27 Nov. 2013. <http://www.kotex.com/na/articles-info/preparing-for-your-first-mammogram/50109>.

The Origami of Heartache

"I want my money back," said the customer in the rumpled cashmere coat. She shoved the grocery bag of gaily-wrapped presents at the employees manning the store's help desk.

The trainee froze. The unlined skin around his eyes paled with fright. He looked at the woman standing next to him. Her badge read, 'Hello, I'm Angela, your manager today.' She signaled with a small tilt of her head, "Get the reason for the return."

The trainee continued to stare at his supervisor. Angela shoved his arm. The trainee jerked his head then rolled his eyes while sing-songing the words, "Don't want to do this."

"You were employed to do this," said Angela, not looking at her trainee.

"You just take them now," said the customer. She looked at the two of them but thrust the bag towards the male trainee. The presents rustled and throbbed.

Deliberately, Angela turned away from the interaction to watch another counter where an employee smoothly rang up sales. Her trainee twisted and turned, searching for possible escape routes.

"Take them. Take. Them." The customer was drawing the store's attention. The boy fumbled under the counter and tape rolls fell one after another onto the floor. Angela glared at him.

"What are you doing?"

"I'm looking for the return form," he said through gritted teeth. Red splotches bloomed on his neck. Like an agitated chicken, once, twice, three times his head jerked forward and back before stopping to perch precariously on his neck.

"Why are you returning these items?"

The customer slammed the bag onto the floor, hunched over the counter to get within inches of his face.

"Why does anybody need a reason? Isn't it enough I don't want them?"

Eyes wide, the trainee put some distance between them and whipped around to tap Angela on the shoulder. Arching a plucked eyebrow, Angela shook her brown helmet of hair.

"Make her happy," she whispered before looking away from the counter.

"The store needs a reason or we can't take them back," he said. His voice trembled with fear or annoyance, at one woman or both.

The woman rocked back and forth on her feet. Heel to toe as the clock in the store ticked on. She picked up the bag. Presents rattled as she swung the bag like a pendulum. The trainee watched without breathing. Angela felt his trance. She fought the urge to look back.

"You want the reason?"

The boy tensed. Angela wondered if he was going to cry or run away.

"I told him I had to have a biopsy and he said he didn't love me, had never loved me, and there was always something missing. Now which 'return' category does that fall under? Wrong size? Wrong color? Wrong price? Broken-hearted?"

Angela clamped her hand down on his arm to keep him there. "It's good experience," she rationalized.

The trainee cleared his throat, opened his mouth, and cleared his throat again. The woman stared at him, then abruptly leaned over the counter, closing the distance between them. She bared her teeth.

"You're saying—if I don't have a good enough reason, you won't take them back?" She kept her gaze on the boy. Her voice grew louder. "That's not what it said on the receipt." The trainee was crying now. The woman rummaged around in her handbag.

Angela, in her navy Henley, pressed kakis and unscuffed nurses' clogs, decided she had to step in.

"I can handle this. Give me the form." The trainee shoved the return form into Angela's hand almost knocking her down. He slid out from behind the counter, picking up more speed until he reached the Men's Room. He disappeared.

Angela turned to the customer with a mouth set in the practiced half smile of those who hold power. With the modulated tones of many in-service trainings, she asked, "How can I help you?"

"You can give me my money back. All of it." The customer swatted some dirty hair out of her eyes. "Look I know I have the receipt in here," she said, her hand digging deep into her purse. Scraps of tissues, wads of paper and various bits of debris spilled onto the counter.

A crowd of customers was watching, grumbling, shifting their weight from side to side. Employees were shaking their heads and whispering. Angela swept the spilled contents of the purse into a box grabbed from under the counter. She firmly grasped the woman's arm, turning her away from the gawkers.

"Let's just get the formalities out of the way so you can get your money back." Angela's voice was low. Demeanor nonjudgmental. Her face soft—like the Buddha of retail.

"I told you, I have the receipt. You have to give my money back." The woman's gait hesitated.

Angela wanted to keep her moving. She was embarrassed for the woman thinking she might dump all the belongings in the purse onto the floor.

"Why are you pushing me?"

"We want to do everything we can to make you happy with our store." Angela droned on in the soothing voice she had used this morning with her husband to avoid their usual pre-work fight. She propelled them both onward towards the loneliest corner in the store. The woman tripped over a box of tie downs.

"You're not listening to me," the woman hissed as Angela tidied the buckled ribbons.

"Oh but I am, " and Angela took the woman's arm again and they journeyed towards the noiseless gloom at the back.

The woman looked over her shoulder at the swarm of busy people at the front of the store. Her shoulders slumped.

"Just take them. I don't even care about the money at this point." Her features dissolved with each step into the darkness. The woman's grip loosened on the grocery bag. Angela just had time to grab the bag of presents before it hit the ground.

"I can't 'just take them' back. We have to fill out the form whether you get your money back or not." Angela emphasized little groups of words hoping the woman would get with the program. What a way to start the day. In the woman's hurt look, she saw again the pained face of her son as he waited for the ritualized sniping and all out war of most mornings. No wonder he was having a hard time in school. No wonder she was getting called on the carpet for her abrupt treatment of employees.

She handed the bag back to the woman, carefully rearranged her face into an expressionless mask then took a deep breath.

"People are looking. It's the holidays. I'm sure you want to get this done so you can go home to your family." Angela laid her hand on the woman's arm with what she hoped was reassurance and compassion.

"I don't give a rat's ass 'it's the holidays,'" said the woman and pulled her arm away jangling the presents. "My husband lied to me for months but you think I'm taking up too much of your time. That's rich."

"I just need to match the merchandise against the receipt. Fill out the form. That's all. A formality."

Angela's impatience was carefully hidden. She got them going again, walking into the back of the store, past the last few customers and into the eerie silence of the kayaking department. Angela stopped them by two camp seats. The woman looked very small and fragile. Long boats were hanging above their head with placards warning boaters to wear their personal flotation devices, or life preservers, at all times near or on the water. Different lengths and weights of paddles were pinned to the walls like dead butterflies. The woman's mouth opened as she looked around. Gently, Angela pressed a camp seat against the woman's leg hoping she would take the hint.

"You want to make sure you got all the presents out of

your house, don't you?"

The woman narrowed her eyes. The pupils dilated then shone with tears. She crumpled down into the camp seat. The metal frame groaned with the sudden weight.

"You have to unwrap the presents." Angela stood behind the adjacent camp seat.

"I don't want to unwrap them. They were gifts I bought for him and his children." The woman's sullen contrariness echoed Angela's husband's mood hours ago. Her hands throbbed.

"You've still got to do it. It's like pulling off a band aide. Let's get this over with so you can move on." Angela consciously loosened her hands' grasp on the seat.

"You keep hurrying me. Why? The store's almost empty now." The customer sucked her teeth. The pretend wood of the boat hulls amplified the sound. Angela looked around to see if the woman was correct. She let out a long sigh. Carefully, the woman took each wrapped gift out of the grocery bag and laid it on the floor in front of their feet. Angela grew impatient again. Her hands tightening and shoulders squaring for a fight.

The gifts blinked in the light. Their happy decorations of tissue paper, curly ribbons, and tiny balls of silver, red, and green threw bizarre shadows against the boats, paddles and holiday decorations. Angela stared back at the Help Desk suddenly feeling as unhinged as she had this morning.

"Okay, we'll mark 'other' as the reason for returning the items."

"But it's not 'other.' He was deliberate. For months he told me he loved me then he took it back."

"I don't understand," said Angela looking down at her wedding ring.

"Like I said. I told him about the test results. My doctor said they needed to do a biopsy. He denied he ever loved me. He took back his love. Said I wasn't enough. My love wasn't enough. Our love was defective." The woman ran out of breath. The silence gobbled up all the in-service trainings, soothing phrases and polished expressions.

"Sounds like he was trying to be hurtful."

The woman watched Angela worry the gold circle on her left hand. The skin was wrinkled and pale underneath.

"He did hurt me. That's why I want my money back. At least."

"Like I said, we just need to match the items to the receipt. It'll just take a minute."

"You don't get it. You don't sound like you want to get it. You're just like him." The woman pushed back the same dirty hair to better glare at Angela.

"She's right," Angela thought. "I don't want to hear. I want this over."

The woman picked up a small oblong gift decorated in

golden teddy bears stamped on a green background. She carefully placed her nail under the tape and broke the seal. A boy's tee shirt fell out of the paper to cling to her knees. "He has an eight year old son. His son would come up and put his head on my chest. Snuggle up to me. He ran back to give me a hug when his mother, the ex-wife, picked him up." The woman held the tee against her face.

Angela reached for the item.

"Life is good," the woman read as she gave it over.

Angela professionally folded the boy's tee into a small square, ready to be stacked with all the other tees in the store. The woman picked up the wrappings and folded them into a neat square, plain side out. Angela drummed her fingers along the chair top.

"You're upset. Do you have someone you can call?"

"No. You said this would be good for me. So we're doing this." A muscle in the woman's jaw fluttered.

Angela sighed, swiveling her head around to see the sun-faced clock on the wall. The tee shirt was checked off the receipt and started the pile of returned items.

The woman picked up a box of dancing stars imprinted on fragile tissues and decorated with a lacy silver bow. The bow jangled with handcrafted earrings.

"Wait. I don't see earrings on the list."

"These are mine. My first earrings. Originally my mother's first earrings. To be his daughter's first earrings.

They're not from your store," she said untying the filigreed silver earbobs from the ribbon trim. "He had a daughter by his first wife. The girl was always cold and never had on socks with her sneakers. I showed her this website. Good clothes and shoes for teenagers. We bookmarked the boots she wanted. I was to buy her socks to go with the boots. But by the time her father went to buy the boots, they were sold out. So I got her the sweater instead of socks." She handed the red sweater to the manager and pocketed the earrings.

"Make sure you don't lose your earrings. They could fall out of your coat." Angela imagined her pretty dark-haired daughter, looking so much like her husband, same frowns, same disdain for her, in the deep red sweater and silver earrings. "The sweater's very pretty. I'm sure his daughter would have liked it. I can see my daughter wearing that sweater." Angela sat down from the weight of the image.

"Thank you. I loved his children." The woman balled up the tissue paper.

"Yes, I can tell. They're thoughtful gifts."

Angela was surprised when the woman threw the wadded wrappings into a red kayak suspended in the air above them. "They'll never find it up there," she thought. The sweater went into the pile of returned items.

"I'm so lost." The woman was crying softly. Angela closed her eyes to keep back her tears. She pulled an undershirt from a nearby rack and offered it to the woman.

"Blow your nose on this. It's okay. I'm the manager. Let's keep going."

The woman wiped her face—blew her nose on the undershirt and handed it back to Angela. The woman picked up a stiff package of plain gold paper. She undid its red string to show a book on camping in the Appalachians.

"We picked up his son from university. Good school. Good son but his father was mad at him for the usual adolescent things. Being late, disorganized, unsure. But his father was good, yeah, good and mad, scowling, uncommunicative. No talking for the four-hour ride home. I tried to break the silence. Read funny stories. He just got madder and madder. The son got quieter and quieter." The woman tried to blow her nose on the wrapping paper. "It's no good," she said shredding the paper in wild uneven strips.

Angela winced with each screech of the paper.

"There's just one more item."

The woman rubbed the indentation in her lip for a beat. She smiled and Angela glimpsed the attractive woman of a month ago.

The last package rustled as it was turned over and over in the woman's hands. It changed shape with each movement. The two women's chests rose and fell together. The woman gave the package to Angela.

"You do it."

Angela felt the compact weight of the gift and immediately knew what it contained. Like the woman, she slid her nail under the tape and slipped the soft inner gift from the store's distinctive stiff paper. She dropped the outer layer to the floor. Without the harsh confines of the paper, the fragile inner tissue paper burst open. An expensive North Face coat exploded onto Angela's lap. Shaking out the coat, Angela saw her husband's present lying unopened under their tree. Gasping she said, "I picked the same coat – different color, for my husband." Tears formed in the corners of her eyes.

They smiled in recognition of shared purchases.

Angela began folding the coat to add to the pile of returns. One of the store's silly little knitted hats was stuffed into the coat's left pocket.

"He's left handed." The woman shook out the hat embellished with two interlocking hearts on the band. "We were planning a ski vacation. He's losing a little hair. I wanted his head to be warm."

Angela thought back to vacations where she had squabbled with her husband. On their first vacation, she had learned of their unexpected pregnancy. He had been less than thrilled with the morning sickness. On another vacation, they had spent most of their time at the Emergency Room as the doctor set their son's broken arm. There was a happy time eating mangoes during the wait for their daughter's birth. Another trip, nothing extraordinary, just out of sorts. Each vacation catalogued and weighed in her mind. The woman interrupted Angela's thoughts.

"I bought them the morning before they called."

"You bought – the hat? What? Who called?" Angela avoided looking at the woman by wadding the wrapping papers into a ball.

"The doctor's office called to say they found calcifications on my mammogram. They said it was a significant." The woman paused. Angela noticed she was folding and unfolding the papers. The woman closed her eyes and swayed. She bit her lips. "A significant area, and I needed to schedule the biopsy, a needle biopsy with a breast surgeon. The office gave me some names of breast surgeons."

"You don't have to tell me this." Angela unfolded the papers, smoothed the creases, and folded them again. The origami of heartache.

"Don't you want to hear how this ends?" said the woman.

The manager blinked. Her hands gathered the wrapping papers into a ball. "It's not necessary." The papers expanded into a loose hodgepodge of colors and textures.

"But it is. I came home from work that night. Don't know how I got through the day. He poured us our usual glass of wine. Talked about the kids and plans for the holidays as I wondered how to tell him. Christmas was only four days away. I told him how excited I was to be celebrating the holidays with him and his family. What I had planned for meals for the kids and for us. He smiled and said it was so good to have me with him. That he loved me."

Angela knocked over her seat in her haste to discard the used wrappings but there was no place to put them. The woman was crying.

"I told him I had something to tell him. It wasn't a big deal but I was a little anxious and so might be quieter than usual." The woman stopped moving. Stopped crying. "Quiet on and off. I told him I had to have a biopsy. I lied."

"You lied?" Angela avoided the woman's eyes by righting her chair.

"Yes, I told him the biopsy was not a big deal. Should I have told him?"

"I don't know." Angela wondered how many secrets she had kept from her husband and how many he had kept from her. She remembered the postpartum haze and the series of fights ending with sleepless nights, crying babies, and the growing disenchantment. Their clumsy attempts at reconnection calming down into a settled but detached arrangement. And the hidden bank account.

"It was a big deal. They would do another mammogram to guide the insertion of a needle so they could get a sample." The woman's face tightened with pain and fright.

Angela was drawn into the scene. "What did your husband say?"

"At first he just sat there. Then he changed. A light switched off inside him. He turned away. Got up to pour another glass of wine. He looked everywhere but at me. He said he didn't love me. He had never loved me. That there had always been something missing and he couldn't be with me through this."

Angela looked down at the mangled wad of wrappings in her hands.

"When I asked why, he said his late wife had been very sick for a long time and he couldn't see himself helping me like he helped her. I sat there stunned, looking at this man I loved, had loved. Then he got up and left. Just left. No word. No anything. Left his own house." The woman finished her indictment with the guttural sound of grief – head back, mouth stretched, primal, rising up from the wet muck of need.

Angela's hands covered her mouth smothering her urge to join the howl – centuries of female rage and disgust. She leaned over to lay her hand on the woman's knee, increasing the pressure of her fingers until the entire palm settled on the woman's leg. The woman bobbed rhythmically. Angela's body joined. Their beings united. Angela felt the wrappings slide out of her hand into her lap.

She ran the hand up and down her breastbone, feeling for the heartbeat.

"Can you forgive him?"

"No." The woman stopped rocking.

Sudden laughter from the front of the store caught their attention. Angela threw the ball of wrapping papers and tissues into the same red boat as the woman had earlier. It bounced around scattering decorations throughout the life preserver section.

"I do get it." Angela helped the woman from her chair. "We'll leave this for the boy to clean up." They walked to the cash register. Angela totaled up the amounts and handed the woman her money.

"I'm so sorry."

The woman crumpled the bills in her hands.

"The biopsy was negative. The doctor called it a false positive and I should be happy to find out it was nothing," she said stuffing the money into her pocket to join the hammered heart earrings.

The Origami of Heartache

A study completed in 2012 estimated the rate of overdiagnosis of breast cancer was 1.3 million in the last 30 years. Overall, studies suggest that 15% to 30% of cancers may be overdiagnosed. Overdiagnosis is defined as:

- the diagnosis of a condition or disease, especially cancer, more often than it is present, or
- the diagnosis of a disease such as cancer that will never cause symptoms or death over a patient's lifetime.

Overdiagnosis of cancer does not take into consideration the rate of progression of the cancer in causing problems for the person. Cancer can have a fast, slow, very slow or non-progressive rate. Overdiagnosis can inaccurately inflate the survival rate of a disease or cancer without accurately reflecting the actual health benefits of treatments.

Mammograms can produce false positive results (indicating a change or problem in the breast when it is not present) or false negative results (missing a true change or problem in the breast). False positive results lead to significant psychological stress, the use of invasive medical tests, possibly unnecessary treatments, surgery and the risks of complications even deaths. In the last decade, studies show the annual rate of false positives range from 5% to 15% of mammogram patients costing the US over

$100 million annually. Distressingly, "over a 10-year period, between 30% and 50% of women screened every 1-2 years can expect a false-positive result, and between 7% and 20% receive a false-positive biopsy recommendation." Another study concluded that with a decade of annual mammography screening, the majority of women (61%) will receive a false positive result and one in twelve will be referred for biopsy. Biopsies increase medical costs for the patient, are inconvenient, create anxiety and pain, produce scarring, and disrupt or sever relationships.

False positive results impact patients' probability of returning for future mammograms. Patients who have a false positive result from mammography, with further imaging procedures to rule out cancer, are less likely than the general population to return for future screenings. Patients who have a false positive and go on to have an invasive medical procedure to rule out cancer are even less likely than the above group to return for future screenings. Shifting the screening times from every one to every two years reduced a woman's chance of a false positive by one third and did not make a significant difference in the diagnostic rate of late stage cancer diagnosis.

While overdiagnosis and false positive errors are different concepts, one study found a connection between the concepts. Researchers followed "vulnerable women" for six years beyond an initial screening mammogram. In the study, "vulnerable women" were defined as patients with lower educational levels, belonging to racial/ethnic minorities, having limited incomes, and a rural residence (not by the patients' medical characteristics). Vulnerable women were associated with a greater rate of false positives and a medical facility's propensity to overdiagnose. Researchers suggested a bias in a set of facilities over a six-year period based on beliefs of the "vulnerable" women's lesser likelihood to follow-up with medical tests and their higher cancer prevalence than in the general population (see the article by Goldman, 2011).

Mammography has a false negative or missed cancer rate of at least 8 to 10 percent due to technology error (machine and technician/radiologist), dense breast tissue (especially found in breasts of people under 50) and the similar appearances of normal and cancerous tissue. Having a mammogram read independently by two radiologists significantly decreases the false negative rate.

While false mammography results have layers of costs to the patient, the medical community and the country's economy, the partners and families of the patients, the "cosurvivors" (the newly coined term for partners of seriously sick patients), are impacted also. Some women chose not to tell their partners about their routine/screening mammography, further diagnostic testing, or biopsy results, hoping to avoid scaring their partners and families. Under this strain, new or young romantic relationships tend to break up easier than relationships with a longer history. Married women labeled as "seriously ill" are six times more likely to have their male partners leave them becoming separated or divorced than a married man with a similar diagnosis (see the article by Parker-Pope, 2009).

Male cosurvivors leave medically ill women for a variety of reasons.

- Men can be intimidated and unprepared for the role of caregiver to a sick wife, partner, or family member.
- Men tend to have smaller social networks than women and with the added responsibilities of caregiving can become emotionally and physically isolated.
- Workplaces have been less aware and less supportive of men's caregiving for their women.
- Men are less emotionally resilient than women – they have more difficulty adapting to stressful situations than women.
- Paradoxically, men leave sick partners because of their fear of abandonment by women.

Organizations are being created to help cosurvivors gain the necessary knowledge and skills for caregiving while specifically guiding and reinforcing men's efforts in this area.

Supporting a partner through a serious medical illness is acknowledged as a large determinant of a woman's quality of life and the quality of care and treatment protocol she receives. In a study of brain tumor patients, divorced or separated patients were more likely to be hospitalized, less likely to receive and complete treatment regimens from standard medical care to clinical trials, and more likely to die at home (Glantz, et. al., 2009). Scientifically rigorous research on the impact of divorce and separation on breast cancer victims is needed.

In summary, overdiagnosis and false positive results from medical testing are different concepts but have similar harmful effects.

	Overdiagnosis	False Positive
Concern	Irrelevant diagnosis	False alarm
Harms		
Physical	physical effects of unnecessary diagnosis/treatment with morbidity and mortality risks	discomfort/ complication from invasive diagnostic tests
Psychological	labeled and increased sense of vulnerability	anxiety and relational aftermath
Economic	cost of treatment with health insurance label of pre-existing condition impacting ability to obtain insurance and increasing health insurance premiums	cost of diagnostic testing
Relational	disruption of relationships abandonment of patient	disruption of relationships abandonment of patient

References:

Berg, Wendie A. "Tailored Supplemental Screening for Breast Cancer: What Now and What Next?" *American Journal of Roentgenology* 192.2 (2009): 390-299. *American Roentgen Ray Society.* Web. 27 Nov. 2013. <http://www.ajronline.org/doi/abs/10.2214/AJR.08.1706>.

Brooks, Megan. "An Equalizer for One Racial Disparity in Breast Cancer." *Medscape Multispecialty.* Medscape Medical News, 3 Oct. 2012. Web. 30 Dec. 2012. <http://www.medscape.com/viewarticle/772016>.

"Can Breast Cancer Be Found Early?" *American Cancer Society: The Official Sponsor of Birthdays.* American Cancer Society, 24 Oct. 2013. Web. 26 Oct. 2013. <http://www.cancer.org/cancer/breastcancer/detailedguide/breast-cancer-detection>.

Cancer Statistics Working Group. "US Cancer Statistics 1999-2009 Incidence and Mortality Web-based Report." *Department of Health and Human Services.* CDC, Prevention, National cancer Institute, 20 Mar. 2013. Web. 27 Sept. 2013. <www.cdc.gov/uscs>.

Carney, P A., T. A. Bogart, B. M. Geller, S. Haneuse, K. Kerlikowske, D. S. Buist, R. Smith, R. Rosenberg, B. C. Yankaskas, T. Onega, and D. L. Miglioretti. "Association between Time Spent Interpreting, Level of Confidence, and Accuracy of Screening Mammography." *American Journal of Roentgenology* 198.4 (2012): 970-978. *MedPub.gov*. Web. 16 Jan. 2013. <http://www.ncbi.nlm.nih.gov/pubmed/22451568>.

Eitan, Amir, Philippe L. Bedard, Alberto Ocana, and Bostjan Seruga. "Benefits and Harms of Detecting Clinically Occult Breast Cancer." *Medscape Multispecialty*. Medscape Medical News, 2012. Web. 1 Jan. 2013. <http://www.medscape.com/viewarticle/773537_6>.

Fernandez, Elizabeth. "High Rate of False-Positives with Annual Mammogram." *UCSF: Advancing Health Worldwide*. Ucsf.edu, 17 Oct. 2011. Web. 16 Jan. 2013.

Friedenson, Bernard. "Is Mammography Indicated for Women with Defective BRCA Genes? Implications of Recent Scientific Advances for the Diagnosis, Treatment, and Prevention of Hereditary Breast

Cancer." *Medscape Multispecialty*. Medscape, 9 Mar. 2000. Web. 2 Jan. 2013. <http://www.medscape.com/viewarticle/408048>.

Glantz, Michael J., Marc C. Chamberlain, Qin Liu, Chung-Cheng Hsieh, Keith R. Richards, Alixis Van Horn, and Lawrence Recht. "Gender Disparity in the Rate of Partner Abandonment in Patients with Serious Medical Illness." *Cancer* 115.22 (2009): 5237-5242. *Wiley*. Web. 2 Jan. 2013. <http://onlinelibrary.wiley.com/store/10.1002/cncr.24577/asset/24577_ftp.pdf;jsessionid=88CF4860C714025BD633B6A04A878E7D.f02t01?v=1&t=hn97b233&s=d0c30eab9ef3ed73cee373c47522d17e58dd4d6f>.

Goldman, L E., R. Walker, D. L. Miglioretti, R. Smith-Bindman, K. Kerlikowske, and National Cancer Institute Breast Cancer Surveillance Consortium. "Accuracy of Diagnostic Mammography at Facilities Serving Vulnerable Women." *Medical Care* 49.1 (2011): 67-75. *MedPub*. Web. 16 Jan. 2013. <http://www.ncbi.nlm.nih.gov/pubmed/20966780>.

Grabler, P, D. Dupuy, J. Rai, S. Bernstein, and D. Ansell. "Regular Screening Mammography before the Diagnosis of Breast Cancer Reduces Black:

White Breast Cancer Differences and Modifies Negative Biological Prognostic Factors." *Breast Cancer Research Treatment* 135.1 (2012): 549-553. *National Center for Biotechnology Information.* Web. 26 Oct. 2013. <http://www.ncbi.nlm.nih.gov/pubmed/22886477>.

Huynh, P T., A. M. Jarolimek, and S. Daye. "The False-Negative Mammogram." *RadioGraphics* 18.9 (1998): 1137-1154. *radiographics.rsna.org.* Web. 1 Jan. 2013.

Magnus, M C., M. Ping, M. M. Shen, J. Bourgeois, and J. H. Magnus. "Effectiveness of Mammography Screening in Reducing Breast Cancer Mortality in Women Aged 39-49: A Meta-Analysis." *Journal of Womens Health* 20.6 (2011): 845-852. *National Center for Biotechnology Information.* Web. 2 Jan. 2013. <http://www.ncbi.nlm.nih.gov/pubmed/21413892>.

"Mammography." *Wikipedia: The Free Encyclopedia.* Wikimedia Foundation, Inc., 2013. Web. 26 Oct. 2013. <http://en.wikipedia.org/wiki/Mammography>.

Parker-Pope, Tara. "Divorce Risk Higher when Wife Gets Sick." *The New York Times* [New York] 12 Nov. 2009: n. pag. Print.

"Type I and Type II Errors." *Wikipedia: The Free Encyclopedia*. Wikimedia Foundation, Inc., 2013. Web. 26 Nov. 2013. <http://en.wikipedia.org/wiki/Type_I_and_type_II_errors>.

Activity 1

If you are female, describe the steps of a breast self-exam (BSE).

> Do you do a BSE monthly or occasionally or never?
>
> What encourages you to do it?
>
> What discourages you?

If you are male, describe the steps of a testicular self-exam (TSE).

> Do you do a TSE monthly or occasionally or never?
>
> What encourages you to do it?
>
> What discourages you?

Have you ever felt a lump/abnormality? If so, what did you do? If you have not felt a lump/abnormality, what would you like to believe you would do?

Activity 2

Draw your breasts or testicles.

> If alone, describe them to yourself in the mirror.
>
> If you are with someone, describe them to that person.
>
> If you are in a group, show your drawing and describe them to the group.

How did you feel about doing this? Proud? Embarrassed? Shy? Militant? What do you know about yourself from this – doing the exercise and listening to another person?

Activity 3

In triads containing at least one man and one woman, rotate through these six situations. Role-playing each situation for 10 minutes then discussing with the observing third person what happened, how it felt, and what you learned.

Situation 1: A female person describes to her/his partner their cancer history. The third person calls time at 10 minutes sharing what she/he observes.

Situation 2: A male person describes to her/his partner their cancer history. The third person calls time at 10 minutes sharing what she/he observes.

Situation 3: A female describes getting a call back for another test after the radiologist spots an abnormal or suspicious spot on a mammogram. The third person calls time at 10 minutes sharing what she/he observes.

Situation 4: A male describes getting a call back for another test after the radiologist spots an abnormal or suspicious spot on a mammogram. The third person calls time at 10 minutes sharing what she/he observes.

Situation 5: A female has to go in for a routine mammogram. She decides not to tell her partner but he finds out she went in for testing. The third person calls time at 10 minutes sharing what she/he observes.

Situation 6: A female has to go in for a routine mammogram. She decides to tell her partner. The third person calls time at 10 minutes sharing what she/he observes.

Resources:

"Angelina Jolie Has Double Mastectomy Due to Cancer Gene." *BBC News: US & Canada*. BBC, 14 May 2013. Web. 15 May 2013.

Bryan, Meredith. "Why are These Men Leaving Their Wives? The Reasons behind Husbands Leaving Their Seriously Ill Spouses to Face Illness Alone." *Women's Health*. Oprah, Aug. 2011. Web. 1 Jan. 2013. <http://www.oprah.com/relationships/Why-Men-Leave-Sick-Wives-Facing-Illness-Alone-Couples-and-Cancer>.

"The Couples Survival Guide." Oprah, Aug. 2011. Web. 1 Jan. 2013.

Jolie, Angelina. "My Medical Choice." *The New York Times* [Los Angeles] 14 May 2013: n. pag. Web. 15 May 2013.

"Sharing Your Feelings About Cancer." National Cancer Institute at the National Institutes of Health. Web. 8 Nov. 2012. <http://www.cancer.gov/cancertopics/takingtime/page4>.

"Talking with Your Friends and Relatives about Your Cancer." *American Cancer Society: The Official Sponsor of Birthdays*. American Cancer Society, 30 May 2013. Web. 26 Aug. 2013. <http://www.cancer.org/treatment/understandingyourdiagnosis/talkingaboutcancer/talking-with-friends-and-relatives-about-your-cancer>.

Renovation

The epiphany had started innocently enough with her choice of dress. Lina discarded a red hot number with a handkerchief hem and spaghetti straps, then a leopard print that hugged in all the animal places and the flouncy black number that twirled up.

She removed a deep purple dress from its plastic Lord & Taylor shroud. It had a cowl neckline held up with teensy little cords that dangled then plunged to a vee at the base of her butt. *Maybe he needs an invitation to riot*, she thought.

She tried on the dress. It looked great from the back. *Still got the back.* With a deep breath, she turned to face herself head-on in the mirror. A full frontal image. She gasped.

"Oh no, I'm a fixer upper," she wailed.

When was the last time I wore this dress? It's can't have been more than three years ago? She leaned forward so her tears would fall onto the carpet and not on her dress. She looked at her back again. Sucked in as much air as she could and did a Doris Day pose. Her breasts were definitely in a different place than three years ago.

Crap. Crapppp. When did gravity hit? I missed the memo. She lifted up her breasts.

Hmmm. Too high. Cleavage under the chin. Either I'm an aging celebrity showing off her plastic surgery or a

Dallas Cowboy cheerleader. Not what I'm going for.

She let the bad breasts drop. She pushed them up, just a little, going for somewhere approximately mid-chest. "Okay, this works," she said aloud to the mirror.

Guess I need a brassiere. I need the Golden Gate of Bras.

Groping through her underwear drawer, she pulled out the well-used boned strapless. Shook it into shape. *The suspension bridge. It'd show in the back.* She let the bra drop to the floor.

She examined another bra with clear plastic straps that crisscrossed at the waist. *Never could breathe in this.* She had a flash of instruments of torture from the Inquisition.

A couple of tangled bras hit the ground. They landed in vaguely breast-like disarray. The cups stayed perky, taunting her with their perfect shapes. *Spackle.*

She pulled out more bras, fitted them against her chest, and let them drift down to the floor. *Ugh. It's like fall in the land of bras.* She giggled. *Or Home Depot for breasts … I am losing it.*

At last, she found the backless bra from the heap on the carpet. Two cups that attached to her body with double stick tape on side tabs. She rummaged for the adhesive tapes. *Duct tape by Maidenform.* Undergarments sprayed half in and half out of the drawer. *It's got to be in here somewhere.*

In the middle of the quest, her best friend Cybil telephoned. "When are you going to the party?"

"As soon as I duct tape myself into this dress," Lina replied, the piles of lace and elastic decorating her feet.

"What?"

"Oh you know. It's one of those strapless-backless contraptions that needs its own ... sticky tab thingies." Lacey straps snagged her feet. Her brain hooked on clasps.

"Are you sure that's a good idea? Duct tape. Sounds painful and what if the tape unsticks?"

"It's awful. Really truly awful."

"Okay then, I'm not seeing why you need to do this?"

"I've got to do this."

"Tell me why?

"My breasts droop."

"Yeah, well, we're not 25 anymore. So ..."

"I need this bra to work. And it needs sticky tab thingies to hold up and sometimes they unstick."

"Sounds like you have experience with the unsticking. So why are you willing to chance it? The unsticking I mean?"

"The unsticking is embarrassing, painful. But it usually doesn't usually happen. Not if you don't move too much, don't sweat, and don't stand by a steam table. Pray it's not humid tonight." Lina pointed her toes and shook the ankle free of mess.

"That's a lot of don'ts. Who are you trying to impress and are you sure your breasts are the best enticement?"

"I'm trying to impress this … guy," she said. A fuchsia bra hugged the other foot, snarling around her big toe, hiding the chipped nail polish on the other toes.

"Yeah, well I didn't think you were changing teams in the middle … "

There was a pause in the conversation. Lina's attention was wrapped around the bra. After a few beat, she got the phone balanced between ear and shoulder. "And well, no. Not really sure about the breasts but they're all I've got to work with." Lina's hands were finally free to cup her breasts into the right position. She let go of her breasts. The disappointing boobs slipped down her chest. "If I lean over just right, get the bra placed just so, the tabs will stick for three to four hours. It should be okay." Her voice quavered. A large furrow appeared on her brow. "If I'm taped by nine, we have to leave the place by one at the latest, preferably midnight."

"Or you turn into a pumpkin. I'm coming over Ms. Vanity Fair. I've got to see this," said Cybil hanging up.

With one foot struggling in the Sargasso Sea of underthings, Lina was still standing, mentally constipated, when the doorbell rang. Shaking her foot free, she ran down the stairs in her bikinis to hide behind the door.

"Welcome to lingerie hell."

Cybil shut the door and looked at her almost naked friend. Her friend's first words were, "Girl, your breasts look fine to me but hey I'm not a man. Fantasies of perky grapefruit halves never did much for me."

"Gravity. I'm being attacked by gravity. We need to shore up my foundation."

Cybil followed Lina upstairs.

"And they're uneven. My left boob is way bigger than my right."

"That's true of everyone by physiology. That I know," Cybil said with a sigh.

"And they have veins. No one in Playboy has veins."

"Don't you want your boobs to have circulation? No circulation—they get gangrene and fall off."

"I just want to be pretty tonight," said Lina.

"Yeah and the only thing you have to offer is your looks, specifically your breasts."

Cybil surveyed the room to avoid watching her friend melt down. The multicolored, multi-fabric shapes cascaded out of the dresser, one bra neatly stacked on the top, falling in clouds on the floor to froth like the milk on a latte—frilly black, demure white, girlish pink, screaming red and classic navy. "It looks like a bra graveyard."

Holding up a battered and dingy beige bra, straps held in place with a safety pin, Cybil said, "This one needs a burial."

"Give it back. That's my favorite. Always fits, always looks good, doesn't pinch or ride up. Of course, the manufacturer discontinued it," and Lina snatched it out of Cybil's hand.

"Looks like an eight year olds' double slingshot," said Cybil. She snorted while mimicking taking a pot shot at the nearby wall.

Lina raised her eyebrow at Cybil. Cybil shook her head. Lina frowned. She spoke to the bra in the overly sweet, singsong voice of a woman to her lover, "Don't listen to that nasty woman. She doesn't care that my boobs hang low and they wobble too and fro – without you. I'll never give you up." Smiling, she kissed the old bra before putting it front and forward, the place of honor, on top of the dresser. But the frown reappeared as she continued the search. "This is the bra I was talking about," she said waving the backless/strapless contraption overhead like a cream-colored flag of dating surrender.

"It looks like a weapon of mass distraction. So you can't move in it?" Cybil sat down on the bed.

"Not too much."

"I have to ask. What happens if you move too much?"

"Last Christmas, I wore this backless dress to a party. Under the mistletoe, my date took me in his arms, buried his nose in my neck and got his sweater caught on my earring. We were hopping about in circles trying to untangle ourselves with our heads cocked to one side. Attracting a crowd. The romantic moment was totally lost." She shuddered. "With a sudden movement, I managed to jerk my earring loose. Breaking it. Something falls on my foot. We look down. My bra has landed. I kick the bra under the table. Smile at my date. Mission accomplished.

But the bra lands on this woman's foot. She shrieks, reaches down and raises the damn thing in the air and bellows, 'Whose is this?' Some guy laughed and yelled, 'What is that?' I looked away. My date looked at me. Then followed a weird discussion about 'to bra or not to bra.'

My date smirked and asked if I had any more fun planned for the evening or would we be improvising? At which point, he moved in for a quick feel. I might have giggled, tapped my foot and told him 'turn around was fair play.' We both laughed and people stared at us—putting two and two together. The woman gave me back my bra after every one signed it."

Lina sat down next to Cybil on the bed. "Did you know gel ink is impervious to hand washing?" Lina's hands were white from effort. Cybil wrestled the bra from her friend's clutching fingers.

"Okay, so a little embarrassing. What happened to the date?"

"He disappeared into the second date black hole with the next day's email. 'Had fun but looking for a different fit'."

"Ooh-hoh. He gets points for a humorous letdown."

"Not funny."

"Is so." Cybil patted her friend's hand. "What happens if you sweat in this press-on bra?"

"It sticks forever, like a frustrated stalker, like sand in your crack, like insurance points, a computer virus, or a leech. Let me tell you, sweat is this bra's superglue."

"Really? Superglue? Looks like a normal piece of fabric to me."

"Not so, my innocent friend. After some hot and heavy flirting on a third date, different guy, I went to the bathroom to remove the bra." She flapped her arms against the sides of her ribs, cradling a breast in the crook of each elbow and continued, "Said I had to powder my nose. In the bathroom I tried to peel off the bra. I may have let out some tiny little screams as I tore layers of skin off my boobs. Ended up needing to fix my eye makeup from the tears of pain. Restaurant-goers ogled as I left the Ladies Room. My date had already paid the check by the time I reached the table minus the layer of breast skin. I winced getting into his car. He looked annoyed. Later, he said, 'Your chest looks like ground chuck.' I was tearing up – it hurt so much. He continued, 'And I'm a vegetarian.' To sum up that neophyte relationship, I spent the rest of the night alone with a bag of frozen peas on my naked chest. Looking at the ceiling and wondering whether I should paint it beige like all good

Jewish girls."

Cybil took the bra from Lina to better examine it.

"It looks innocent enough." Cybil turned it around and around looking for an explanation.

"Oh but it isn't. It's from the Inquisition, I'm sure of it."

"Okay, so the million dollar question, what happens at the steam table?"

"The bra droops. The cups droop. The adhesive pulls the skin from your ribs around to the front. Everything slides forward and down. The Titanic of bras. Every breast for themselves. No life boats on this ship. Or like a facelift gone wrong. Tight in all the wrong places. Wrinkled, sagging and buckling in other places. And it happens without warning. One minute you're perky and popular, the next you're droopy and alone. Men are morbidly fascinated but not aroused. You can hear them mentally saying, 'Exactly how old is she? Maybe we should start a fund for a boob job. Can't she get some gel padding?' Which sloshes by the way. Bad idea. One compassionate date said, 'You should see someone about that. Aren't you kind of young for a dowager's hump?' as I hunched over. I've given up Chinese. And buffets."

"Maybe you should go braless?" Cybil said. "It's not like you're a double D."

"No," and Lina leaned over, held her breath, positioned the breasts in the bra, and stuck the tapes to her unsuspecting skin. Slowly, she stood up and took a tiny sip of air. "Hhhh. I blame Victoria's Secret for setting unrealistic expectations of perpetually perky breasts." Her voice was small and high like she had been inhaling Helium. Her ribcage didn't move and the dress settled onto her body. "Don't just stand there. Get me a towel. Remember, I can't sweat."

"Move or eat Dim Sum," was Cybil's snippy reply. "Forget I said that. Everyone will be mesmerized by the way your breasts defy gravity."

"You think this is funny but it's very important," Lina said. Her face red from the effort of not doing – breathing, sweating, moving her arms. She shuffled towards the stairs.

Cybil picked up the scattered bones from the bra graveyard—stacked them neatly to go back into the drawer. When she picked up the favorite oldie, she shook her head before placing back on the top of the dresser. Going downstairs, Cybil saw her friend standing by the door eerily still, breathing slightly, a battery-operated fan whirling in front of her chest.

"Oh good grief. Why the obsession with this bra?"

"Well something's got to stick to me and it sure hasn't been the men."

Cybil deliberately blocked the door. Lina's eyes darted then drooped. Her mouth went slack. She took on the air of a dejected dog, loved once, played with, petted, to become the fixture in the corner, almost forgotten, sagging with years. Tolerated in an offhand way. Cybil could not bear to see her friend give up. She pressed.

"Slick easy answer. Not buying it. Tell me – what's behind the obsession with your breasts?"

"Well I want the easy answer. It's too hard to do this – try to date, grow old, get passed over for younger women, prettier women, women with perfect breasts. Men judge women by their breasts. Women, even women notice. And judge. My breasts aren't perfect. They need renovation. And the only way to renovate boobs is with surgery or the right bra. I won't have surgery but I will pick the perfect bra. Obsess about details. Because the real question is – will I ever be enough as I am?"

Renovation

The concept of a brassiere can be traced back to 2700 BCE but it was not until 1907 when Vogue magazine first used the word *brassiere* in print. In 2010, the average American woman owned nine bras. In the United Kingdom, the average woman owned sixteen bras. Usually, bras are washed every two months.

Bras have become big business. American women buy four bras per year and spend sixteen billion dollars on bras annually. Over the last fifteen years, the average bra size has increased from a 34B to a 36D. The average woman will change bra size six times over her lifetime yet 8 out of 10 women wear the wrong bra size (too big a band and too small a cup size). Despite the average American woman wearing a 36D, most of the fashion world designs for a B cup. A study in 2010 found that 27% of women have decided not to buy an outfit because they did not have the right bra to wear underneath it.

Out of sync with the clothes they can find in stores and wearing bras that are the wrong size, women express difficulty accepting and valuing their breasts and their bodies. When a woman is dissatisfied with her body, usually it comes from two basic, but incorrect, ideas:

1). Bodies can be reshaped into the cultural norms or values by exerting enough effort (exercise, diet, and surgery).

2). Bodies outside of the cultural norms reflect an imperfect woman (such as "I'm lazy" or "She doesn't care about herself or her marriage").

These beliefs create conflicts that can develop into eating disorders, from starving herself to purging behaviors (throwing up, over-exercising, laxative and diuretic abuse) to overeating. A vicious cycle is created of denying food, thinking about the denied food to the point of obsession and possibly purging, feeling awful about yourself and then overeating to comfort the self. Women have moved away from process of attuned eating – eating when a woman is hungry and eating what she is hungry for to the point of consciously and comfortably satiated. Similarly distressing beliefs and behaviors are infiltrating the male population to a significant degree. Billion dollar industries (around exercise, weight loss, and surgical practices) have grown out of this culturally determined body dissatisfaction.

References:

Duenwald, Mary. "Body and Image: One Size Definitely Does Not Fit All." *The New York Times* [New York] 22 June 2003: Health. Web. 4 Jan. 2013. <http://www.nytimes.com/2003/06/22/health/body-and-image-one-size-definitely-does-not-fit-all.html?pagewanted=all&src=pm>.

"History of Bras." *Wikipedia: The Free Encyclopedia*. Wikimedia Foundation, n.d. Web. 1 Jan. 2013.

"History of the Bra." *Xtimeline*. Famento, Inc., 2 Mar. 2008. Web. 1 Jan. 2013.

Lester, Tracey L. "How Many Bras Do You Own?" *Glamour: Fashion: Dressed*. Glamour, 1 May 2009. Web. 1 Jan. 2013. <http://www.glamour.com/fashion/blogs/dressed/2009/05/how-many-bras-do-you-have.html>.

Lester, Tracey L. "Psst ... What do You Think Your Bra Size Is? (Chances Are, You're Wrong)." *Glamour: Fashion: Dressed*. Glamour, 9 Apr. 2009. Web. 1 Jan. 2013. <http://www.glamour.com/fashion/blogs/dressed/2009/04/psstwhat-do-you-think-your-bra.html>.

"Victoria's Secret: 6 Surprising Bra Stats." *Redbook* (n.d.): n. pag. *Hearst Women's Network*. Web. 1 Jan. 2013. <http://www.redbookmag.com/beauty-fashion/tips-advice/fun-bra-facts#slide-1>.

Zernike, Kate. "Sizing Up America: Signs of Expansion From Head to Toe." *The New York Times* 1 Mar. 200: n. pag. Web. 21 Nov. 2012.

Activity 1

Divide a flip chart, whiteboard or chalkboard into two columns, one for female and one for male. Write your responses to these questions.

If you are a woman, describe your favorite bra.

    What makes it your favorite?

    How many bras do you buy every year?

    What is the average price of the bras?

    How much do you spend each year on bras?

    What do you think about this number? Is this how you want to use this money?

    What is your response to taking off your bra? What do you feel and think?

If you are a man, would you wear a man's bra? (In the US, they are called a 'compression vest,' 'compression bra,' 'manssiere,' 'gynecomastia vest,' or 'the bro.' In Japan, they are called 'men bras.')

    Why do you or would you want to wear a bra?

    How many bras would you or do you buy every year?

    What is the average price of the bras?

    How much do you spend each year on bras?

    What do you think about this number? Is this how you want to use this money?

    What is your response to taking off your bra? What do you feel and think?

After discussing these points, answer the following questions:

Would you wear a push-up bra, minimizer bra, or gel/water bra?

What do you think of women who wear these bras?

What do you think of men who wear bras?

How many bras do you own (or your partner or mother/father or sister/brother)?

What is the total dollar amount for the number of bras you own (or your partner or mother/father or sister/brother)?

What do you think about using money for this purpose?

Activity 2

If you could wave a magic wand and change your breasts, would you change them?

How would they look, feel, smell, and/or taste different?

What do you think the changes would get you?

What is holding you back from making these changes?

Activity 3

Individually, divide a piece of paper into 3 parts.

In the first part, write down the reasons a person may want breast implants.

In the second part, write down the reasons a person may want breast reduction.

In the third part, write down the reasons a person may want breast reconstruction.

Fold the paper in half and then again (into fourths) for anonymity.

Gather up the papers and write out the three categories (Implants, Reduction, Reconstruction) along the top of a chalkboard or whiteboard.

From the gathered papers, write out the lists of reasons for each of the three categories.

For each of the categories, underneath the list of reasons, write out the beliefs and feelings that are the basis for the list.

For each of the categories, underneath the list of reasons then the lists of beliefs and feelings, write out the industries that support and/or are created from the top two lists.

So what do you know about yourself, your peers, and society's values?

Resources:

www.85b.org/bra_calc.php. (International Bra Size Calculator. No nonsense and easiest calculator of your bra sizes in different countries' sizes)

www.gynecomastia.org (has resources for male breast apparel)

JustBreastImplants. "A Breast Augmentation Patient Education Resource." JustBreastImplants.com, Web. 26 Sept. 2013.

www.underworks.com (has many different options for men wanting/needing a male bra/compression shirt)

Major Department stores have fitters from their bra departments and during special times, from the major bra makers – Wacoal, Donna Karan, Calvin Klein.

The Rose Garden

The dog rambled into the room. He circled his bed a couple of times, pawing at it, rearranging the padding, then with a long exhale eased himself down near the very center. His heavy head lolled off the side. The long tricolored ears splayed out. Yellowed eyes rolled up. As the old dog started to snore, they resettled their attention on each other. Raj sighed. Tamara wrapped the sheet tighter around her body before returning to the attack.

"The In Case of Emergency info's in a file on my laptop. I call it, This Sucks."

"Very funny."

"Well I knew it had to be done."

"I was going to do it tonight."

"No you weren't. I'll bring a copy of the file with me tomorrow."

"It presupposes some events."

"Yeah like I'd die."

"Yeah like that."

"Or I end up in a coma from the anesthesia."

"Or that."

"Could happen ... "

"I wish you wouldn't do this."

"Dying would leave you free."

"What do you mean by that?"

"That you could move in with your ... Twinkie." Tamara twitched her nose at Raj. It was a gesture he had once found endearing but now forewarned a battle.

"Don't call her that."

"I've always called her that."

"No, you didn't. She was our friend."

"No, she was your assistant."

"And our friend."

"Not calling her 'friend' any more. Twinkie. She'll be the 'Twinkie' now!"

"Not nice."

"It's not the time to be nice. We've run out of nice time, big boy. Let's put it on the table."

"I don't want to do that tonight."

"Tell me Raj, tell me when would be a better time. When I'm dead or in a coma or throwing up from the chemo and radiation. Yeah, let's do it tomorrow. Right after surgery. Right after I have my breasts cut off. Tomorrow."

"Don't ... "

"No. Now. It's now or never for us."

"Tamara, I love you."

"You didn't always. You ate a ... Twinkie."

"I can't do this now. I am drowning."

"But we have to. Now."

In the corner, the sleeping dog murmured. His grumblings were loud enough to interrupt the couple. Then his sudden howl jarred them.

"Talk to me. Be honest with me. For once."

"We went through two years of counseling. Wasn't that enough? Our life is good. We are good."

"Life is good for you. Did you forget I have surgery tomorrow? Like you conveniently forgot all those years – collecting your precious awards, moving up and away from me."

"No I, I didn't ... forget."

"Right. Well tomorrow morning at 7:30—I'm going to have my breasts cut off. Deal with it. It changes everything."

"No it doesn't."

"Don't be an idiot. Of course it does. You said you were a breast man. You tell people you fell in love with the All-American girl who laughed all the time. Big breasts and long blonde hair. I am going to lose it all. Look at me. See me. Now imagine me different."

"Tamara, I can't bear imagining you different."

"Bear it. Use your creative vision."

"Tamara, if I start, I won't be able to stop imagining you different."

"Then tell me what you see. Tell me you won't be different."

"Today, tomorrow, all the tomorrows. I want to see you as the girl I fell in love with. In that gallery."

"Oh please. Don't pretend you love me."

"Tamara, listen. I'm trying to love you. Remember … "

"No I can't remember feeling that you loved me. It was so long ago."

"Yes it was long ago but I can still feel the heat. I'm reminded every August."

"Wasn't that when you fucked 'Twinkie'?"

"No. That was winter. There weren't any flowers. This is the day we met. Late summer."

"Okay. Okay. It was so hot. The air conditioning broke. I had to open all the windows in the gallery." Tamara scratched her head and the sheet slid.

"And you were the hottest thing in that gallery."

"And you thought you were so cool. Checking out all the nudes. Looking down my dress. Probably other girls' dresses."

"No, no others. Only your dress. It was a great dress."

"I got rid of it when I learned about the affair."

"Oh? I loved that dress."

"That was a long ass time ago."

"I fell in love with you in that dress. I wish you had kept the dress."

"It stood for everything you threw away. I cut it up with your favorite scissors. Left it in the bin by your pile of Art Director magazines. Even cut up your magazines. Ruined your scissors. You didn't say anything. You didn't notice."

"My many sins—not saying that I noticed."

"Your greatest strengths. Not saying. Not noticing."

"I miss you in that dress."

"Well it wouldn't fit anymore." Tamara swaddled herself in the sheet – hugging her arms to her chest.

Raj felt himself congealing, everything becoming stuck. Stone-like. Shaking himself, like the old dog would do after a long sleep, he asked the forbidden question.

"If you knew about the affair, why did you wait so long to confront me?"

"I was waiting for you tell me. Why is it my job to be your conscience? Why can't you grow up?"

"Because I'm a fool. You are the one perfect thing I have in my life. And I fucked it up."

"Yeah and tomorrow I won't be perfect. That you'll notice. Deal with it."

Tamara spat the last sentence at Raj. Raj looked around for something to do. He began gathering debris on the bed—the pictures of surgical reconstructions, office visit slips, pens and markers. Tamara watched him. The dog pawed, chasing imaginary squirrels, teeth grinding in effort.

"Do you have to snipe at me? Can't we have a good night?"

Raj arched his back all the way into his neck. Forehead creases deepened. Cords of muscle in his thighs and belly grew taut spreading out into his arms, clenching his fists. He stretched his mouth open to shriek. Tamara shook her head slowly. Before he knew what he was doing, Raj threw the markers in his hand across the room. They hit with mini explosions causing the careworn dog to howl in outrage. Tamara jumped before turning back to accuse Raj.

"A good night. When's the last time we had a good night?"

The startled dog huffed before limping from the room. The sudden movements, the noise, frightened him. The dog was old, fifteen years old. Old as their marriage. Showing some wear and tear as he aged. Like they did. Like their marriage. Raj sagged with exhaustion. Feeling for the bed like an old man, blind, every joint aching, he sat on the bed and held out his hand for Tamara to join him. Without touching him, she sat down. The tangled sheets and blankets formed a valley between their bodies. Tamara smoothed the space by tucking the sheets deeply under her legs.

"I don't know how to have a good night now. So much has happened and so much is going to happen. It's like a machine that's turned on and can't stop. How do we stop it? Why aren't you there for me?"

"I'm trying to do my part. Remember with me. Please. For the love of God, let's try to piece it back together. I want to be there with you. I want to love you again. I want you to stay with me."

Tamara moved closer to hold Raj's face in her hands.

He started to squirm away but she held him tight. His sounds of distress started out small then grew, becoming wails of grief and impotence.

"For once, stay with me when it gets tough."

"I don't want you to leave me."

"I don't trust you to stay."

"Please don't leave me. Go back to that night in the garden behind the gallery. Where we met."

They heard the dog moving around in the other room. His soft irregular shifts of weight amplified by the wooden floors as he weaved around furniture, searching among their home's rooms.

"How will this help?"

"I need the memories to … "

"Remind you of why you thought you loved me?"

"No, to put in place all that has happened to us. To make some sense of things. To have a context for tomorrow."

"Don't you think it's too late?"

"I don't know, I don't know. But I have to try."

"Whatever." The dog was silent in the other room. "We drank some wine, talked, ate some leftover bread and cheese."

"But it started then. We were so in love."

"Maybe."

"I saw you sitting by a wall covered with rose vines.

The roses framed you."

"The wall was damp. My dress got stained with the moss."

"The dress was pink almost red. Your hair had come undone. Strands fell into your eyes when you talked."

Tamara opened her mouth for the usual denial. She gulped in some air. Her face grew flat then questioning.

"I remember you pushing my hair back behind my ears."

"You had these big gold hoops on. And bright red lipstick. Your mouth was luscious. As my mother used to say, like a peony."

Tamara looked at him. Raj could see her confusion.

"How do you remember all this?"

"I remember the night smelled of roses. My mother had this perfume she would wear – Shalimar – and it was like the roses gave off Shalimar."

"My mama wore that too."

"Do you remember the wine?"

"God it was awful. Some French red. Unpronounceable."

"We laughed."

"You dribbled wine."

"Which you pointed out."

"You had breadcrumbs in your beard. I wiped away the crumbs."

"I was so surprised you touched me."

"I had to touch you and you didn't look away."

"I couldn't look away. I wanted you so bad."

A gentle rhythmic snoring came from the other room. Raj shaped his hand to the curve of Tamara's neck. He continued.

"With that look, I knew I would love you."

Tamara took Raj's hand from her neck. She traced the lines on the palm.

"You were so mysterious with your turban. Foreign. Almost scary."

"I couldn't believe it – I found myself unwinding my turban."

"Why did you?"

"I don't really know … "

"Your hair was long and thick. Blue black."

"I wanted to show you something private, something beautiful."

"It was like a long rope I wanted to wrap around my wrist."

"To bind us together?"

"May-be." The word was two syllables in Tamara's mouth. "It was sexier than anything anyone's every shown me."

"It must have been the perfumed night."

"No, no it was more than that."

"I showed you my hair because I needed … to … make you look at me with wanting."

"Well that you got. We kissed … goodnight. You rubbed your chest against mine. I was embarrassed and aroused. Tingling."

"It was hard to let you go."

"It was hard to go."

Tamara tried to give his hand back to him but Raj gripped hers tight. They heard the dog get up and start to prowl again. Traveling through the rooms. Probably looking for something to eat. Scraps dropped on the floor since it wasn't his dinnertime.

"Why did you cut your hair?"

"I was no longer worthy, not pure or wise. I cut it out of disgrace."

"You never told me this."

"You never asked. Tell me the truth. Why didn't you ask when I cut my hair?"

Tamara pulled her hand away from Raj.

"I didn't want to know."

Raj gathered her hand back to him.

Tamara looked away as she spoke. "Why did you stop wanting me?"

"I don't know. I can't wrap my mind around what I did. How I hurt you. How I hurt me. What I did to us."

"How did we get so lost?"

"All I know is that when I think of you, I smell roses, I see roses, I go back to that night in the garden. But I can't see you. Maybe I lost the image, lost the picture. Maybe I thought some other woman would give me back my rose garden."

"Did she? Did she smell of gardens? What flower did she remind you of?"

"She didn't. You are my flower."

"A Venus flytrap?"

"Tiger lily. But it's like I got lost in a maze and kept looking for a way out. Only to go deeper and deeper. I needed you to pull me out I was in so deep."

"But you walked into that maze. When I think of you all I see is your betrayal. My garden has thorns and bare earth. Like the lines of the surgeon. No flowers."

"I am unclean. I am so sorry. I am so sorry."

"Can you see me as the girl you fell in love with?"

"I don't know how."

"Make me that flower again."

Raj rocked and keened. Wailing out his failures. Stealthily, drawn by the distress, their dog peeked through the door. All four paws planted, the dog stared at them and bayed with the urgency used to alert them of approaching sirens. Having done his duty, the dog left the room.

"Crazy old hound dog." Tamara said.

"This is shit. I can't fix it."

"Try. Try hard."

Raj collected the markers strewn on the floor, matching brightly colored caps to their proper pens. With his artist's hands, Raj smoothed Tamara's body into a reluctant canvas. Using a marker the verdant green of the first spring leaves, he drew a gentle line from the tip of her right collarbone to her sternum. With other markers, he added roses of peach, yellow, and creamy ivory against the olive of her skin. Buds, tightly closed, some almost open, the first blooms, the fully opened flowers almost overpowering in their glory, sharing all – swollen with pollen, dewy, juicy with their fertility.

Raj smiled for the first time that day. He picked up a rosy hued marker to draw another spray of tight pink buds that started on the left collarbone to journey across her chest ending at the delicate shelf where hard ribs blended into soft belly.

Tamara started to laugh. "You drew my dress."

"Yes. From that night."

"Will you grow your hair out? Wear a turban again?"

Raj didn't answer. Instead, he drew and drew until her body was a lush garden, roses, petals, leafy vines and swaying stems trailing from collarbones to hips until the surgeon's lines become insignificant twigs in the lush landscape.

"Did you keep any of my turbans?"

"Yes. The orange one—for wisdom."

Raj frowned. He drew tiny thorns among the flower heads. Scatterings of seedpods appeared around her navel. Flung open under its own weight, a flower lost its petal. For a second, their noses lifted, searching for fragrances of flowers past, pulling them together. They sniffed old dog and Betadine.

"I am more afraid you will leave me than I'll lose my breasts."

Raj knew he had to say something to keep her with him. His hands trembled.

With the shuffling gait of a creature at ease with himself and the world, the dog ambled back into the room to bay once before waiting expectantly at the side of the bed. One ear was notched from a fight long ago, his snout was grey, but the dog's worn fur comforted Raj.

"What about my dog?"

"I'll take care of our dog."

Raj ran his hand down the battered ear. The dog watched and listened, finally settling down to warm their feet.

The Rose Garden

Cancer rates are on the rise in the US. Over a lifetime, one in three women and one in two men will be diagnosed with cancer. Breast cancer rates are rising also. From 2008 to 2020, the number of breast cancer cases is estimated to increase by 26% with 80% of patients surviving over 10 years. In 2012, U.S. breast cancer statistics predict about 1 in 8 women will develop invasive breast cancer in her lifetime. One in a 1000 men will develop breast cancer in his lifetime. The estimated diagnosis rate of new breast cancer cases for American women in 2012 is 226,870 and for men it's 2,190. For diagnosed women, approximately 28% or 63,300 cases of breast cancer will be the non-invasive earliest form of breast cancer. The most significant risk factors for breast cancer are being a woman and growing older. In 2011, the U.S. had 2.6 million breast cancer survivors with a quarter of a million survivors less than 40 years of age.

Breast cancer is the most commonly diagnosed form of cancer (around 30%) among American women. Breast cancer is the second highest cause of cancer death in women after lung cancer. Improvements in detection and treatment have brought the overall death rate to 3% for women (1 in 36). In 2012, the estimated deaths from breast cancer for women were 39,510 and for men were 410.

Mastectomy, the removal of one or both breasts

with or without removal of the lymph nodes, is a surgical treatment for breast cancer. In 2008, 78,000 mastectomies were performed in the U.S. There are four categories of mastectomies – modified radical mastectomy, simple-total mastectomy, skin-sparing mastectomy, and nipple-sparing mastectomy. In some treatment centers, such as the Mayo Clinic in Rochester, NY, mastectomy rates have dropped from 45% of breast cancer patients in 1997 to 30% in 2003 but have risen to 44/43% in 2005/2006. An MRI (magnetic resonance imaging) performed preoperatively is correlated with an increased rate of mastectomy surgery. Some women choose to have smaller surgeries, lumpectomies, where a part of the breast, instead of the whole breast, is removed. There is evidence of repeated surgeries after lumpectomy. One in five women in the U.K. will have another breast surgery after their initial lumpectomy. More women are choosing to have their non-cancerous breast removed along with the identified cancerous breast up from 2% in 2000 to 6% in 2006.

The Women's Health and Cancer Rights Act of 1998 for all 50 U.S. states mandates insurers cover the cost of breast reconstruction but seven out of 10 women are unaware of their options for breast reconstruction after mastectomy. 89% of women want to see what results look like before making a decision and less than one-fifth of mastectomy patients will go on to have breast reconstruction. In 2011, over 96,000 breast reconstruction procedures were performed in the U.S. Some reconstruction may be done at the same time as the mastectomy, but other women may need to postpone reconstruction due to the demands of radiation treatment, the stage of the breast cancer, the need to return to work and home responsibilities, and the insurance/health-care costs.

References:

American Cancer Society. "What are the Key Statistics about Breast Cancer?" *What is Breast Cancer?*. American Cancer Society: The Official Sponsor of Birthdays, 1 Oct. 2013. Web. 26 Oct. 2013. <http://www.cancer.org/cancer/breastcancer/detailedguide/breast-cancer-key-statistics>.

American Society of Plastic Surgeons, and The Plastic Surgery Foundation. "Breast Reconstruction Information." *BRA Day USA: Closing the loop on Breast Cancer.* 2012 Breast Reconstruction Awareness Day, 2012. Web. 26 Oct. 2013. <http://www.bradayusa.org/breast-reconstruction.html>.

GlaxoSmithKline Oncology. "When We All Stand Up, Cancer Will Stand Down." *We All Stand Up/weallstandup.com*. GlaxoSmithKline Oncology, 16 Jan. 2011. Web. 1 Jan. 2013. <http://us.gsk.com/html/healthcare/healthcare-we-all-stand-up.html>.

Harding, Anne. "Mastectomy Rates Still Declining across U.S." *Reuters* [New York] 14 June 2010: n. pag. *Reutersreprints*. Web. 13 Jan. 2013. <http://www.reuters.com/article/2010/06/14/us-mastectomy-rates-idUSTRE65D5TS20100614>.

Katipamula, R, T. L. Hoskin, J. C. Boughey, A. C. Degnim, C. S. Grant, K. R. Brandt, C. L. Loprinzi, S. Pruthi, and M. P. Goetz. "Trends in Mastectomy rates at the Mayo Clinic Rochester: Effects of Surgical Year and Preoperative Magnetic Resonance Imaging." *Journal of Clinical Oncology* 27.25 (2008): n. pag. *jco.ascopubs.org*. Web. 18 Jan. 2013. <http://jco.ascopubs.org/content/27/25/4082.full.pdf>.

Mulcahy, Nick. "Advanced breast Cancer in Young American Women: On the Rise?" *Medscape Multispecialty*. Medscape Medical News, 26 Feb. 2013. Web. 4 Mar. 2013. <http://www.medscape.com/viewarticle/779917>.

Salahi, Lara. "Breast Cancer Patients Opting for Lumpectomy or Partial Mastectomy Might Need 2nd Surgery, Says Study." *abcnews.go.com*. ABC News Internet Ventures, 12 July 2012. Web. 13 Jan. 2013.

Surveillance Epidemiology and End Results. "SEER Stat Fact Sheets: Breast cancer." *National Cancer Institute*. National Institutes of Health, US Department of Health and Human Services, Apr. 2013. Web. 26 Sept. 2013. <http://seer.cancer.gov/statfacts/html/breast.html>.

"U.S. Breast Cancer Statistics." Breastcancer.org,
    14 Mar. 2012. Web. 1 Jan. 2013. <http://www.
    breastcancer.org/symptoms/understand_bc/statistics>.

www.weallstandup.com. (GlaxoSmithKline Oncology)

Activity 1

Take a picture of your breasts (nude or in a tight tee shirt) and print out several copies. Imagine a design for your breasts or a design that incorporates your breasts.

Transfer the design onto the picture. What is your response?

Using body paint, transfer the design onto your bare breasts or the tight tee shirt. What is your response?

Using body paint, have another person paint your breasts with the design. What are your responses?

Activity 2

If you were having a double mastectomy tomorrow, what words or symbols would you put on your breasts before you went in for surgery?

Why did you choose those particular words?

What are the feelings that contributed to picking those words or symbols?

What are the thoughts that contributed to picking those words or symbols?

Activity 3

On the Internet, find pictures of double mastectomies, single mastectomies, lumpectomies, and breast reconstructions.

How would you choose between the options of double mastectomy, single mastectomy, lumpectomy, breast reconstruction, or declining medical treatment?

Would you have the nipple tattooed back on (a 15 minute procedure)?

What would you miss most after mastectomy?

Is reconstruction worth the time, pain and resources to you?

What would you do/feel/think if your partner elected to use prosthetics?

What would you do/feel/think if your partner chose not to use breast reconstruction surgeries?

Resources:

www.bradayusa.org

Brandenburg, D L., A. K. Matthews, T. P. Johnson, and T. L. Hughes. "Breast Cancer Risk and Screening: A Comparison of Lesbian and Heterosexual Women." *Women Health* 45.4 (2007): 109-30. Web. 6 May 2013.

"Cancer Facts for Lesbians and Bisexual Women." *American Cancer Society: The Official Sponsor of Birthdays*. N.p., n.d. Web. 6 May 2013.

Garcia, Michelle. "Health: Health and Treatment: New Breast Health Rules Leave Out the Lesbians." *The Advocate* 17 Nov. 2009: n. pag. *Here Media*. Web. 6 May 2013. <http://www.advocate.com/health/health-and-treatments/2009/11/17/new-breast-health-rules-leave-out-lesbians>.

"Lesbian, Gay and Bisexual Women." *Susan G. Komen*. Susan G. Komen, 2013. Web. 6 May 2013. <http://ww5.komen.org/BreastCancer/Statistics.html#lesbian>.

Orenstein, Peggy. "Our Feel-Good War on Breast Cancer." *The New York Times* 28 Apr. 2013: Sunday Magazine. Web. 29 Apr. 2013.

Parker-Pope, Tara. "Facing Cancer, a Stark Choice." *The New York Times* [New York] 21 Jan. 2013: n. pag. Print.

www.rexhealth.com (website with comprehensive information about cancer treatment options)

www.rightactionforwomen.org (Christina Applegate Foundation for information and financial assistance for breast cancer screening and treatment)

Surveillance Epidemiology and End Results. "SEER Stat Fact Sheets: Breast cancer." *National Cancer Institute*. National Institutes of Health, US Department of Health and Human Services, Apr. 2013. Web. 26 Sept. 2013. <http://seer.cancer.gov/statfacts/html/breast.html>.

www.weallstandup.com (GlaxoSmithKline Oncology)

A Collection of Forks

"Put on your best bra and get your breasts out there. It's time to date. What's the worst that can happen?" Mary said.

"Well I could get my heart broken again," Linda moaned to her best friend.

"Not all men are shits," Mary had said from the complacency of her decades long marriage. "We'll get you some pictures, exaggerate a few things, hope for someone with bad eyesight."

"Nice. Thanks for the support." Linda looked at her hands wondering when the veins had appeared so prominently. It was probably during the year of separating from her husband and the three years of apprenticing herself to a nunnery, as she called the post-divorce period. "Probably should tell you – I have a date this weekend."

"You're shitting me."

"Really good support there, Mary. Guess I'm not as incompetent as everyone thinks."

"Including your ex."

"Including all my exes." Linda looked herself over in the deli's window, noting the rows of meat hanging by hooks, little battalions of lifeless chicken, ham and veal. Linda was repelled and fascinated by the similarity of their headless bodies. "So now what do I do?"

Linda's friend took a step back to examine her friend. "Well you've been through Hell and you lost too much weight. You think you should start eating again?"

Linda knew she had lost much in the process. "I've been divorced, widowed, and left at the altar. Even food doesn't stick with me."

"That last ex was kind of mean. Used to creep me out the way he stared at your breasts. I wanted to cover my breasts whenever I was around him. Tell me. Was he weird? Did he slap them?"

"Don't go any further. I'm not answering," Linda interrupted.

'Well no reason to get all huffy. But you did lose a lot of curves. Deliberately?"

"Not going there. But you are right about one thing—I used to be curvy. Where'd the curves go?"

Mary surveyed her friend. "You look fine. We'll get you some breastage at the Pennyrich Bra Patch."

"The what?"

"Pennyrich. You know. They fit you and if we need to, we'll buy you some curves."

"Buy me curves? You mean like padding?"

"More like feats of structural engineering. A suspension bridge with a little gel for shape. The Golden Gate Bridge of bras."

"Nothing like truth in advertising."

"It's dating. There's no expectation of truth for the first three years."

"Won't he be disappointed if, when we take our clothes off?"

"Turn off the lights. They can't tell in the dark."

"I don't know about any of this."

But she had gone with her friend that Saturday to the Pennyrich Bra Patch.

"So what kind of patch is this? Cabbage, rock, bush?"

"Be quiet. Let me get a salesgirl," Mary said and wandered off. Linda looked around. The walls were covered with rows of bras, mainly white and beige durable numbers. Some black and red- still utilitarian looking. Linda had expected colors and lace. A wonderland of frilly things to make her feel young and sexy again. Instead she was in the Ukraine of lingerie.

Mary appeared in front of Linda with a saleswoman in her mid-sixties standing alongside. Mary nudged her friend. Linda stumbled and the saleswoman reached out to steady her.

Mary stepped between the two. "We need help for my friend." Mary gestured in the area of Linda's breasts. "She needs cleavage. Can you do something for her?"

Linda felt the need to explain. "Um, I have a date. The first date in a long time."

"Of course," said the woman.

"I don't want to look ... cheap ... or desperate."

The saleswoman pursed her lips as if concentrating. "Go into the dressing room and take off your shirt."

Linda shot a dirty look at Mary and did as she was told. The curtains didn't close completely as she stood there shivering in her bra, wrapping her arms tightly across her chest.

The saleswoman bustled into the room, laid down three bras, and without hesitation undid Linda's bra. "Yes, I was right. You are a 32C."

Linda tried to cover her breasts. "No I'm not. I've always been a 34B."

"Bodies change. Try this on," the saleswoman handed the bra to Linda. Linda struggled to put on the bra while covering her breasts with her hands.

"My hands will be cold. Bend over," the saleswoman said, not unkindly. Linda leaned over and the saleswoman placed her hands in the bra's cups, jostled things around, and then stood back.

Linda was aghast, mouth open, feeling violated. As warned, the woman's hands were very cold.

Next the saleswoman took two gel packets in the shape of veal cutlets and told Linda to, "Stand up straight while I put these in place."

"What?" The saleswoman took one Crayola Flesh colored gel packet, reached into Linda's bra's cup and stuck the cutlet in. Linda took a step back. The gel cutlet was even colder than the woman's hands. Linda felt unbalanced with the extra perk. The saleswoman steadied her as she inserted the other gel cutlet.

"Look in the mirror."

Linda looked then smiled. "How do I keep them in?"

"They'll conform to your body in a few minutes and stick to you with the heat of your skin. You have to be careful not to move too much or they could migrate."

"Migrate?"

"Well maybe you had placed them underneath for uplift and they could move to the sides. Then you'd have cleavage. Or the opposite, place them for cleavage, move too much, they'll migrate under the breast and you'll get uplift."

"Sure. Noted. No movement when wearing the bra."

"Don't use adhesive or you'll end up pulling the skin off your breasts," the saleswoman warned. They both shuddered. "Just keep your arms by your sides."

"Whatever."

Smiling, they looked at her shapely chest in the mirror. The saleswoman softly patted Linda on the shoulder. Linda flung open the curtains, stuck out her chest, and yodeled into the store, "Mary, Mary, look I have cleavage." The store's patrons stared, six women and three men. A middle-aged man gave her a "thumbs up." The woman beside him whispered into his ear. Linda quickly shut the curtains and a gel cutlet popped out of the bra. "Oops, guess too much movement." The saleswoman handed the flesh colored blob back to Linda. "I'll take the bra in every color you have," she said, "And two packets of the inserts." The saleswoman smiled a saintly smile.

"Well that was right entertaining. Your breastage got a lot of exposure. Probably more than it's had in a while," said Mary cocking an eyebrow.

"Don't be an ass," Linda said shielding her chest with her purchase.

"Wear the red one tomorrow night."

"Yes ma'am. Maybe my husband wouldn't have left me if he had seen me in this get-up." Linda watched Mary steal a quick look at the bras and inserts. "Sure you don't want one?"

Sunday night, Linda strapped herself into the red bra and put in the gel cutlets. It took some maneuvering to get them into place – she was going for not too much uplift and a suggestion of cleavage. And they had to be even. One breast couldn't say "Hi there" more than the other. She broke a sweat. Her breasts looked like over packed grapefruits. She looked at the package the cutlets came in – the resting place for her false advertising and realized she had them on her body upside down. More sweat. When corrected, the cutlets felt cold and foreign lying against her body. Unfamiliar even. But the newly bought curves gave her some well-needed confidence. She put on her three-inch heels and practiced walking with the new center of gravity. Hopefully, the restaurant did not have stairs.

Linda and her date reached the restaurant at the same time. She watched his face fall as he saw her. "Great start," she thought to herself straightening her shoulders. The cutlets pressed against her shirt creating a teeny gap between the buttons. She reached out her hand to greet her date. He opened the restaurant door for her and watched her precede him to their table in the tight skirt. Linda had just enough time to feel self-conscious about the new breasts in her figure hugging clothes. Her date was dressed in the fashionable jeans and layered cotton shirts of the undergraduates she taught. Immediately her date took the seat facing into the restaurant leaving Linda to take the faux rickety chair with her back to the crowd. Was he hiding her, ashamed to be seen with her, or checking out the other entrees? The evening was off to a rocky start.

They looked at each other. "Well, what should we order?" he asked. Linda remembered this as a polite form of 'let's get this show on the road.'

"Wine. I would like a glass of wine," she said.

"Good idea. You like red of course."

"Actually no. Red gives me a headache. The tannins."

"Oh." The waiter appeared. Linda mangled the name

of a wine from the middle of the price range. She watched her date converse with the waiter in French, pausing for adoration and applause. Linda felt compelled to speak.

"Your French is impeccable," she smiled and placed her hands gracefully on the table. He could have been speaking pig Latin for all she knew.

"Yes, I lived there for three years and then brought the woman back with me to New York. We lived together for a year. Then, well, it was regrettable." He looked straight into Linda's face – the same challenge as the nuns in Catholic School. She was being told to behave properly.

Linda's décolleté swelled with the deep breath as she wondered what had happened to the French woman. Did she drown in a vat of red wine, develop a nasal Brooklyn accent, or commit another adequately gauche offence to be exiled back to France? Linda fought the urge to undo the bra tightly binding her breasts.

"What should we eat?" he said purposefully.

"I don't know. It all looks good. What are you getting?" Linda shrugged.

The waiter appeared again. "Can I tell you about our specials?"

Her date smiled at the waiter. "What are your specials?"

The waiter droned on about the three types of oysters, the special mustard the restaurant imported from France, and some kind of sweetbread that sounded illegal and immoral.

"While you don't have my favorite, I haven't had oysters in a while. I want the oysters." Suspiciously like an afterthought, he asked, "Don't you think we should get some oysters?"

Without even waiting for Linda's nod, the waiter said, "Very good choice, sir."

Linda thought, "Oh yeah. Slippery, slimy and an aphrodisiac. I'm excited." Aloud, she said, "That sounds yummy." The waiter caught the edge of the sarcasm.

"Would Madam like something else?" the waiter said using the slightly derisive classification.

"Yes, Madam would like the scallops over lima beans. Thank you." Linda decided to eat and drink well tonight.

With the waiter gone, they talked apathetically about the scarcity of good oysters, the need for butter in French food, and the purpose of sulfites in wine. Time ticked by.

The waiter presented the oysters with a flourish. "St. Edwards Bay. Enjoy," and left them one tiny fork. Linda fought an urge to stab herself in the eye with the utensil.

"What is so amusing?" asked her date.

Linda choked. "Oh, it just looks so lovely."

"Then please take the first oyster."

Linda looked at the offensive bivalves. She took the tiny fork and stabbed the smallest blob, meaning to transfer it to her plate. Her date was watching. He twitched slightly in disapproval. Linda hesitated. Fork in mid-stab. Elbow sticking out.

"You should try the marinade." He mimicked bathing the oyster on its icy shell with the sauce – the ritual dance of the polished and pretentious.

Linda tried to pull the fork out of the offending mollusk. It clung stubbornly to its shell. She applied more muscle and with a jerk of her shoulder inadvertently flung it across the restaurant. It hit the window on her right with a plop and slipped down the glass leaving a trail of edible mucous. "Ick," she thought. "I'm a barbarian." Her date's mouth was open. A waiter quickly wiped the oyster from the window. "I think I'll wait for my scallops."

There was very little talk after the oyster toss. When her scallops came, Linda looked gratefully at two plump circles sitting on a bed of lima beans drizzled with pesto. Picking up a fork, she started to move a scallop onto her plate. "Please have the other one," she said. He looked at her and then looked at her choice of fork. The place settings had three forks. Linda followed childhood rules and started with the first fork on the left but now worried about her choices, the oyster, the fork, the scallop, the date. At this point, the only thing buoyant was Linda's bra.

"Am I not what you expected?"

"No, you are exactly what I expected," said her date.

"Your blouse is open." Linda looked down at the front of her blouse gaping wide and exhibiting a cleavage the size and plumpness of a newborn's bottom, perfectly framed by the red bra. She re-buttoned the blouse and started to saw through the unusually tough scallop. The bed of beans swirled and eddied. Suddenly, a single lima bean, like a rogue flying fish, jumped off the plate and hit her date squarely in the forehead. Unlike the oyster, it stuck. Linda was horrified then awestruck, finally overcome with the absurdity of the night. Her date pressed his lips together and the lima bean fell onto his deliberately rumpled denim. Linda hugged her arms.

"Oh let me get that ... " she started to say.

"No, I think I should clean my own lap," he said. Linda cringed at his frigid tone.

"Alrightey then," Linda returned her attention to her plate.

The waiter appeared. He took away the napkin holding the rogue bean and presented a pristine cloth.

"Would you like anything else tonight?"

"I would like the lentils and garlic sausage," said her date. He looked over at Linda.

"Can I have some bread and butter?"

"Certainly Madam." There was a conspiratorial pause. "May I offer you another glass of wine Madam? For you Monsieur?" They both nodded. The waiter walked into the kitchen, eyes downcast, mouth smirking.

The lentils, sausage and basket of bread appeared followed by a small plate of butterballs. Linda decided to leave the balls for another night and reached for the bread. Things shifted.

"The lentils are divine. You should try some," said her date.

"Thank you," said Linda and looked at her fork collection. The lentils glistened in their oily coating, daring her to eat them. She bravely chose the middle fork wishing very much for a spoon. Lifting some lentils onto her fork, she watched as the mound of slick spheres broke up, slipped through the fork and sprayed the table, rolling hither and yon. Her dated sighed audibly.

"Try the sausage," he said.

"Thank you, I will."

"How do you feel about large sausages?"

"Well, sometimes one can't get one's mouth around them and so they're lonely. Uneaten." Linda recognized a declaration of war, picked up a sharp knife, and purposefully stabbed the largest sausage. Her knife pierced the casing, going right into the center of the meat. A stream of sausage juice leapt across the table. She laughed. "I made your sausage squirt, and now your side of the table is a mess."

"Yes, you have. This seems to have been quite the moveable feast," he said without a smile. No twinkle in his eye, no smirk, absolutely flat. He placed his forearm on the table. Linda watched as the greasy lentils slid his arm out from under him and her date landed face down, perilously close to the tines of his fork.

"Oh my God, you almost lost an eye," Linda leaned forward. Her date put out a hand to keep her away. Linda giggled with embarrassment. Silently, creepily, the waiter appeared with a clean napkin.

"I'm glad my possible disfigurement causes you glee," he said, wiping himself down for a second time that night.

"I'm not laughing at you, mainly at myself, and the absurdity of a first date."

"Well here's something else for you to laugh at," he said with a flat-lipped smile surrounded by a sheen of meaty oil. "For the last hour, you have been sitting here with three breasts."

"I don't understand."

"You have a third breast."

"What?"

"You started out with two breasts and grew a third over dinner," he said pointing to her chest.

"Oh." Linda was pissed. "And your large sausage deflated before it got to be eaten. I'll pop round to the Ladies room," she said. She stood up, slipped on the spilt lentils from earlier in the evening, confined by the tight skirt; she twirled and sat down with a plop in his lap. He was nonplussed as his face bounced off her three breasts.

"You should get the check." Linda was on the verge of hysterical laughter. She planted her feet firmly but didn't know where to put her hands. On his legs, on the faux French table complete with deliberate wobble. Fighting the urge to kiss the top of his bald spot, a little something for the other Sunday night patrons watching their table with mouths open, she tensed the muscles of her legs and rear to hoist herself off him. "Damn you, Mary," she muttered under her breath.

In the ladies room mirror, she saw a pleasantly forty-something year old woman, slender, tallish, with a laughing mouth and in a knit top clinging to three prominences, or maybe two and a half. "Crap," she said and went into the stall to rearrange things. A gel pad had migrated into her newly enhanced cleavage creating a breast bud. Linda thought to herself, forty-three going on twelve, rolled her eyes in imitation of her daughter and removed the new breast. Back at the mirror and without the gel inserts, Linda checked her figure. Her breasts looked just fine. Not overly prominent and not invisible. Another woman joined her. Linda watched the woman apply her lipstick as the young girl next to them blotted her underarms with paper towels. Slowly, Linda walked back to her date.

"I see you've rearranged things," he said.

"Yes, life has a way of rearranging things until we

get it right." Linda slapped down the gel cutlets next to his collection of forks. He looked down at the inserts and then up at her chest. Linda took a deep unbound breath and one by one nailed each cutlet to his side of the table with one of his forks. She smiled. "What fork does one use for filet of asshole?" she asked. His mouth formed a little oh of alarm. She walked out of the restaurant with a remembered sway to her hips.

"Well, how did it go?" asked Mary.

"I can't believe I paid over $250 to be a piece of meat. Do you know where I put the receipt for the Bra Patch?" Linda was planning to return the unused inserts and bras. She had hung the red bra in her closet as a warning.

A Collection of Forks

If you give a teenage boy a dictionary, the word he will most likely look up will be "breasts." Breasts have been a symbol of femininity throughout the ages. As far back as 1500 BCE, Minoan artwork depicts bare female breasts. Breasts fascinate us. Both women and men. In general, women want bigger or different breasts. On average, men tend to like smaller female breasts than woman believe.

Women are acutely aware that young perky breasts are the objects of desire. In general, young breasts are round, firm, and have fullness in the upper quadrants of the breast. Aging breasts are caricatured in the media and a source of industrial inspiration (from lingerie stores such as Victoria's Secret with their push up and gel filled bras promising a youthful silhouette to special décolleté creams and Botox for breast wrinkles to plastic surgery for breast lifts and implants). Over time, breasts may lose firmness, sag downward and spread out giving what is called a "matronly" silhouette. With time, breasts lose fullness in the upper quadrants of the chest and flatten out. The areolas may shrink and change shape. The nipples may turn in. These are normal breast processes beginning in women's forties.

Women's breasts change over their lifetime due to internal and external factors. Most internal factors are the consequence of a change in estrogen level. With the decrease in estrogen levels that comes with approaching menopause, women's breasts become less glandular and fill with more fatty tissue. The connective tissue becomes dehydrated and less elastic. This accounts for some of the changes in the appearance of breasts.

External factors such as environment and lifestyle impact the appearance of breasts. A three year study of identical female twins in Ohio (by plastic surgery residents) concluded that cigarette smoking, drinking alcohol, multiple pregnancies, larger cup sizes, and higher BMI (body mass index) was correlated with less aesthetically attractive breasts (as defined by the plastic surgery residents). Moisturizing the breast skin, hormone replacement therapy after menopause, and breastfeeding was correlated with more attractive breast appearance in the twin study.

In other studies, sudden weight loss and gain is connected with significant changes in breast shape and size. And while going without a bra can be uncomfortable, it is not accepted as a leading contributor to sagging breasts.

References:

American Society for Aesthetic Plastic Surgery. "Twins' Breasts are Revealing: Identical Twin Study Uncovers External Factors that Influence Breast Appearance and Aging." *Press Center: Breast Surgery.* American Society for Aesthetic Plastic Surgery, 4 Sept. 2012. Web. 4 Mar. 2013. <http://www.surgery.org/media/news-releases/twins-breasts-are-revealing>.

Drezin, Martha. "Breaking News: Dos and Don'ts of Breast Aging." *Project Beauty.* American Society for Aesthetic Plastic Surgery, 1 Oct. 2012. Web. 1 Mar. 2013. <http://www.projectbeauty.com/blog/blog-post/breaking-news-dos-and-donts-of-breast-aging/>.

Langan, MD, Michael. "Aging Changes in the Breast." *Medline Plus: Trusted Health Information for You.* U.S. National Library of Medicine, 13 Dec. 2010. Web. 4 Mar. 2013. <www.nim.nih.gov/medlineplus/ency/article/003999.htm>.

Linder, MD, Stuart. "How Does Aging Affect a Woman's Breasts?" *Experts and People.* Sharcare, n.d. Web. 4 Mar. 2013. <http://www.sharecare.com/health/womens-health/how-aging-affect-womans-breasts>.

"Ptosis (Breasts)." *Wikipedia: The Free Encyclopedia.* Wikimedia Foundation, Inc., 2013. Web. 19 Jan. 2013. <http://en.wikipedia.org/wiki/Ptosis_(breasts)>.

Shockney, Lillie D. "What Normal Breast Changes Can I Expect Over My Lifetime?" *Healthy Women: Informed. Empowered.* National Women's Health Resource Center, Inc., n.d. Web. 1 Mar. 2013. <http://www.healthywomen.org/content/ask-expert/1296/normal-breast-changes-over-lifetime>.

Activity 1

Pick up a magazine created for a female audience and a magazine created for a male audience. Tear out all the images of chests, breasts, and torsos.

How are these images used in the print medium?

What are the common characteristics of the images?

Are the images and characteristics from the magazines different for women and men?

Arrange the images from most pleasing to least pleasing to you. Look at your arrangement. How do you define an aesthetically pleasing breast?

Activity 2

In a television interview with William Shatner of the TV series and movie series, "Star Trek," he said that the 1970s TV show could show a breast from the collarbone to just above the nipple but the censors would not allow them to show the underside of a breast (from the crease where the chest wall and breast meet north to the nipple).

1) Design a set of guidelines for showing the breast/chest areas of males and females in a children's show. It should include information about clothes, fabric, erectness of a nipple, tightness of the top, if there are different guidelines for females and males.

2) Design a set of guidelines for showing the breast/chest areas of males and females in a teenager's show. It

should include information about clothes, fabric, erectness of a nipple, tightness of the top, if there are different guidelines for females and males.

3) Design a set of guidelines for showing the breast/chest areas of males and females in an adult's show. It should include information about clothes, fabric, erectness of a nipple, tightness of the top, if there are different guidelines for females and males.

What values are we condoning in our guidelines? Are the three sets of guidelines different and if so, why?

Activity 3

With modeling clay, sculpt the breast or breasts of a 15 year old, 30 year old, 45 year old, and 60 year old.
Line them up side by side.

Describe the models.

What do you feel about each sculpture and about seeing them lined up next to each other?

Resources:

"Breasts." *Wikipedia: The Free Encyclopedia*. Wikimedia Foundation, Inc. 2013. Web. 19 Jan. 2013.

Brooks, Linda, and Jacques Brisson. "Medscape: Medscape Access." *Do Breast Implants Affect Breast Cancer Survival? An Expert Interview with Jacques Brisson, MD, DSc*. Medscape Internal Medicine, 17 July 2013. Web. 26 Oct. 2013. <http://www.medscape.com/viewarticle/807776>.

JustBreastImplants. "A Breast Augmentation Patient Education Resource." www.justbreastimplants.com, Web. 26 Sept. 2013.

www.keep-a-breast.org (youth-focused, global breast cancer website reaching out through art, education, awareness, and action)

Langan, MD, Michael. "Aging Changes in the Breast." *Medline Plus: Trusted Health Information for You*. U.S. National Library of Medicine, 13 Dec. 2010. Web. 4 Mar. 2013. <www.nim.nih.gov/medlineplus/ency/article/003999.htm>.

Got Milk?

"I just got a text about my fun bubbles," said Chanie saluting Becky with her glass of wine.

"Fun bubbles? What's a fun bubble?" asked Becky.

"I wasn't sure. So I looked it up in the Urban Dictionary. Whoa, that was a weird experience. Totally different culture. Fun bubble means breast."

"Who sent you this? A teenager?"

"No, my husband."

"But he's in his fifties." Becky rolled her eyes. "Puerile."

They laughed, lolling around in their stuffed chairs. Glad to be finished with work for the day and out together. Drinks with the girls. A monthly ritual started after college and even continued during pregnancy (non-alcoholic drinks) and the more crazy-making period of child raising (definitely alcoholic drinks).

"Well, what do you call them?" asked Chanie. She untucked her oxford shirt. The stiff fabric floated around her to settle into a shapeless bag on her body.

"Ugh, the ladies," said Becky patting them.

"The ladies? I remember calling them 'The Girls' but now they're 'The Ladies.' Even my breasts have grown middle aged."

"Men still call them melons, casabas, love apples," said Becky. She untied the soft belt at her waist to expose a tiny camisole threaded with burgundy colored ribbons. Becky cupped her heavy harvest. "Ripe fruit.

"Maybe we should give the guys permission to nibble."

"Yeah, right. Nibble would be great, biting not so much. We need another name for them."

They nodded. Sipped. Looking very pleased with themselves.

"The Breast Cancer Society calls them tatas," said Chanie.

"That is so creepy. Why would a health care organization give them a nickname?"

"To make them more touchable?"

"Come here baby, let me reach out and touch your tatas." Becky leered at Chanie.

"Okay, now you're mixing the phone company with the Cancer Society. Eew. Try again."

"My mother used to say, 'Tough titties.' I found that demeaning. Like I was an overcooked piece of steak."

"Moo. What did you call them?"

"My boobies. My first real boyfriend called them that. We were fooling around in the backseat of his Pinto, he lifted up my shirt and said, 'Look at those boobies.' I wanted to throw up. It was tacky. I pulled down my shirt and told him to take me home." Becky pulled her jacket around her chest while Chanie wrapped her arms around her breasts. They grimaced at the memories of teenage scuffles.

"Probably saved you an explosion. Baby batter or the Pinto."

"Hilarious," said Becky.

"As a teenager, I was jealous of girls who developed before me."

"Chanie—everyone developed before you. I used to call you the Mosquito Bite Girl."

"Yeah, I remember—not nice. Hey, at least I could wear a halter and run track."

"Yeah. I, make that my big beautiful tatas, got all this attention. Gawky pimply teenage boys with sweaty hands. Groping me as I passed them on the bus. Feeling me up on dates. Being called a slut by Mosquito Bite Girls like you."

"Hey, I didn't call you a slut. Easy maybe. But not a slut."

"Thanks a bunch. All of a sudden I had these alien tumors on my chest that shifted my center of gravity. At ballet class, I had to bind my breasts. By the end of the year, big patches of skin fell off from the tape. Hurt like hell. I never got my balance back. One of the main reasons I quit dance."

"Ooh. I never knew that."

"Didn't tell anyone. Too embarrassed. We were hormonally stupid."

"And young."

They nodded and Becky continued. "By college, I finally got up enough nerve to wear a tank top, the guys would line up and watch me or more truthfully, watch my breasts. Guys would talk to my breasts. They didn't even notice that my arms couldn't touch my sides from the minimizer bras bought by my mother. My breasts had been relocated to my armpits or squished together for the uniboob look."

"They went from downtown to the suburbs."

"Either place, unnatural."

"That sounds painful. Meanwhile, I spent most of college practically naked trying for any male attention. See my pointy perky breasts, just like a fashion model." Chanie pulled her shoulder blades back and smiled with the perpetually sweet grin of an undersized starlet. "I blame my frozen shoulder on adolescent breast angst."

Both women laughed. Raised their glasses to each other.

"Then came technology," said Becky.

"And wasn't that helpful? Remember when I wore that gel bra to a meeting. Some guy kept asking, 'Where's that sound coming from?' You figured out it was my bra and kicked me under the conference table. Guess I was too close to the problem to hear myself."

"Yep, you sloshed but at least you didn't spring a leak. Remember the poor woman who returned to work too early.

Every time someone had an emotion, said something kind or God forbid sounded in any way like a crying baby, even the door squeaking, she'd run to the bathroom."

"She ruined a lot of shirts with her milk."

"Freaked out the men in the office."

"My breasts never leaked but they do make life interesting," said Becky

"As last night's class will testify. 'Yoo-hoo, Mr. Yoga Instructor! Exactly where do I put my breasts in that pose?'"

"He did look a little cranky with my question."

"Especially when you said, 'Do I put them under my arms? To one side? How do I counterbalance the weight?'"

"Yeah, but the engineer was helpful with the counterbalance issue."

"I think the engineer wanted to get his hands on those love apples of yours. Do some suspension testing."

"Hah hah, very funny. He needs to engineer a supportive line of comfortable bras. Then he can use my breasts as a mold for all I care."

Both of them watched the waitress awkwardly set down their second glasses of wine. She had heavy swaying fruit. Becky shook herself to shift her focus from the probable disaster of boob-flavored wine.

"Chanie, why do you hide your kumquats under so many clothes? You need to take them out to play more often." Becky watched the waitress cantilever herself upright, threatening their wine again before taking off to another table.

"I don't know. It's confusing now I'm a mother. They changed shape when I got pregnant – bigger, fuller, covered with blue veins. They were always in the way. I felt like a cow with udders. Not softly glowing like in the ads. Nursing bras and breast pumps." Chanie shuddered. "Never got used to it even when my breasts went back to some semblance of what they were before nursing."

"Your milk came in. My big breasts didn't work. They didn't leak even when they were supposed to. I felt inadequate. Like God was punishing me for all the fun I had had with them in my youth."

"Becky, I don't think the universe works like that." Chanie smiled down at her breasts. "My daughter used to grab at them with this hungry look in her eyes."

"Feed me, feed me."

"Then my husband would come up behind me to grab and say the same thing."

"Feed me, feed me."

"I lost touch with them literally. Everyone else touched them. They were never mine again."

"Like BB, before babies, when they felt luscious and we bought bras that were about seduction and fun."

"Not about breast feeding and ease of access."

"Yes, the good old days." They smiled wistfully. Sipped

their wine.

"But to feel the mouth of your child," said Chanie.

"Those sharp little teeth—while whacking you with their fists."

"Forget the fists, those little sharp teeth could clamp down. Like I had given birth to a starving gremlin."

"I was jealous you could breast feed. I tried with each of my kids. My milk didn't come in. I wasn't a natural mother according to other women. That I had a psychological problem and chose not to provide for my children. My husband was not so secretly pleased. He said, 'I want them all to myself.' I thought, 'They're mine. You can't have them. You can check them out with your library card for a very short loan period.' I wanted to threaten capital punishment if he kept them beyond the due date."

"My husband alternated between staring when I breast fed and looking away, kind of sheepish."

"At least you didn't have the problems that Cecilia had. After breastfeeding the twins, she would have to roll up her breasts to tuck them into her bra. Didn't she have plastic surgery?"

"Yeah, but in her situation, I could see her point."

"She said they weren't points—they looked more like lawn darts."

"Kinda. She had breasts to her waist. It's like they deflated or something."

"Like they gave up. Maybe in that situation I would have a boob job. Would you?"

"Probably not. I'm a chicken when it comes to surgery and that's no small surgery. A lift and implants. Sometimes you lose sensation. But here's the kicker. She told me about taking off the bandages too early and her nipples fell on the floor." Both women looked down at their breasts.

"Holy shit."

"A toast. Here's to our fun bubbles."

"Maybe we should be drinking milk," and they raised their glasses chest high.

Got Milk?

A quick search of Google provides 56 names for breasts and 400 names for a penis. Going into the website for Urban Dictionary (www.urbandictionary.com) provided more names for breasts but still many times less than the names for a penis. The names for breasts can be positive, friendly, neutral, raunchy and derogatory.

While people can have multiple names for their breasts, the evolutionary function for breasts is to feed our babies. The ability to breastfeed is not dependent on the size of the breasts. Breastfeeding is impacted by many factors including nutrition of the mother, sucking/latching on reflex of the baby, laws and regulations protecting or inhibiting breastfeeding in public, in the workplace, and in child care centers, the availability of lactation specialists to help new mothers, and the promotion/support/hindrance of breastfeeding through public health personnel overlaid with legal, societal, and cultural structures.

In 2010, the Surgeon General's Goal for Healthy People aimed for:

- 75% of women to breastfeed their babies upon discharge from the hospital
- 40% of infants to be exclusively breast fed until at least 3 months of age
- 17% of infants to be exclusively breast fed until at least 6 months of age

- 50% of infants breast fed until at least 6 months of age
- 25% of infants breast fed until at least 12 months of age

A study under the direction of the Centers for Disease Control and Prevention found that by 2010, a significant population of the US was meeting or approaching these goals. Of infants 19 to 35 months old in 2010, four out of fifty US states achieved all five objectives. Overall, the statistics reflect a growing trend towards breastfeeding babies.

- 75% were breast fed at birth
- 33% were exclusively breast fed at 3 months
- 13% were exclusively breast fed at 6 months
- 43% were breast fed at 6 months
- 22% were breast fed at 12 months

In 1991, Unicef, the World Health Organization and other policy makers established a Baby Friendly Hospital Initiative (BFHI) accrediting hospitals that meet a set of 10 regulations. Sweden is considered the global leader in BFHI. In the US, the hospitals on the Pacific coast were the first to comply. The BFHI regulations cover teaching, encouraging, and supporting mothers to breastfeed in hospital, and connecting mothers with resources on discharge from the hospital. Caesarian section delivery has been found to significantly negatively impact the rates and timing of breastfeeding newborns. Other hospital factors impacting breastfeeding rates include the availability of rooming in for the baby with the mother, the cultural values of the mothers, the values and procedures of staff around use of formula and pacifiers, and skin-to-skin contact between the baby and mother immediately after birth.

Inadequate milk supply and discomfort or pain during breastfeeding are the major reasons mothers state they do not breastfeed. Many new mothers report feeling overwhelmed, stressed, and pressured by the issue of whether or not to breastfeed.

References:

Bohling Smith, Pat, Karen Moore, and Liz Peters. "Implementing Baby-Friendly Practices: Strategies for Success." *The American Journal of Maternal/Child Nursing* 37.4 (2012): 228-233. Print.

"Breastfeeding In Public." *Wikipedia: The Free Encyclopedia*. Wikimedia Foundation, Inc., 2013. Web. 4 Jan. 2013. <http://en.wikipedia.org/wiki/Breastfeeding_in_public>.

McKeever, Joyce, and Rose St. Fleur. "Overcoming Barriers to Baby-Friendly Status: One Hospital's Experience." *Journal of Human Lactation* 28.3 (2012): 21-314. Print.

Mollmann, Marianne. "Bloomberg's Breastfeeding Initiative: Let's Start with Paid Parental Leave .." *The Huffington Post* 8 Aug. 2012: Parents. Web. 4 Dec. 2012. <http://www.huffingtonpost.com/marianne-mollmann/breastfeeding_b_1755188.html>.

O'Connor, Mary. "Breastfeeding Benefits & Barriers: Breastfeeding Statistics in the United States." Breastfeedingbasics.org, 1998. Web. 16 Jan. 2013. <http://www.breastfeedingbasics.org/cgi-bin/deliver.cgi/content/Introduction/sta_us.html>.

Quart, Alissa. "The Milk Wars." *The New York Times* 14 July 2012: n. pag. Web. 4 Jan. 2013.

Saint Louis, Catherine. "For the A-Cup Crowd, Minimal Assets are a Plus." *The New York Times* 1 Sept. 2010: n. pag. Web. 1 Jan. 2013.

US Department of Health and Human Services. *Breastfeeding Laws*. National Conference of State Legislatures: HRSA, Maternal and Child Health Bureau, 2011. Web. 4 Jan. 2013. <http://www.ncsl.org/research/health/breastfeeding-state-laws.aspx>.

Activity 1

Give a person a wrapped candy bar. The person is told to hold, unwrap and eat the candy bar with one hand in a bathroom stall.

Could this be similar to having to breastfeed a baby in a bathroom?

(Adapted exercises from Linda J. Smith, BSE, FACCE, IBCLC, 203 Breastfeeding Games)

Activity 2

Take a one yard square piece of fabric. Holding both corners of one side, tie the corners around your neck and arrange the fabric to cover your chest. You have made a primitive "Hooter Hider." Wearing the "Hooter Hider" and holding a baby doll about the same size, weight and softness of a newborn baby, feed the baby using the hooter hider to cover the breast for 10 minutes (usual time needed for a baby to nurse).

Is this comfortable?

Is this easy?

What gets in the way?

What special accessories and support do you need to modify this to fit your body and baby?

What if the baby does not like the "Hooter Hider?"

Do this at your desk at work.

Do this at a fast food restaurant and at a sit down

restaurant.

In each of these situations, notice:

> What is your response?
>
> What are the responses of the people around you?

(Adapted exercises from Linda J. Smith, BSE, FACCE, IBCLC, 203 Breastfeeding Games)

Activity 3

Write down all the names for breasts. Put each name on a different note card. Arrange the cards according to whether the names were:

> Positive
>
> Neutral
>
> Negative

What are the characteristics of the names that are positive, neutral and negative about breasts?

What names would you use with your lover, your mother, your sister, your colleague, and your friend?

Resources

Baby-Friendly USA

http://www.babyfriendlyusa.org

Centers for Disease Control and Prevention

http://www.cdc.gov/breastfeeding

USDA-Food & Nutrition Service Women, Infants and Children (WIC) Program

http://www.fns.usda.gov/wic/

Healthy People 2020, Maternal, Infant and Child

http://www.healthypeople.gov/2020/topicsobjectives2020/objectiveslist.aspx?topic

United States Breastfeeding Committee (USBC)

http://www.usbreastfeeding.org

Beans on a Bus

"Quick, pull my finger!" he said.

"Stop it!" she said.

"You started it."

"What was I thinking?"

"You were thinking beans? On top of a stomach virus … before a twelve hour bus trip?"

Sighing loudly, she rubbed her tummy from one side to the next. He watched her fingers with prominent knuckles and bulging veins pushing the paper-thin skin. The fingers traced a deep concave curve from one hipbone to the other.

Groaning, he tucked the covers tightly around their shoulders. Heads were separated from bodies by eggplant colored sheets of lyocell, dark but not black and the softest least prickly fabric he could find. All at once, her skin had become hypersensitive to sensation and light, a not unusual side effect. They had hoped it would lessen after the treatment was finished but the residual nerve damage caused her to toss and turn at night on their old sheets. So he talked to doctors, nurses and other survivors, researching fabrics, ending up at Bed, Bath and Beyond. He imagined the new sheets cradling her over-worked body, providing comfort, safety, and peace to combat the night terrors of chemotherapy and radiation.

"It wasn't just beans, silly. It was cassoulet. A very

sophisticated recipe."

"Okay French beans and franks with a stomach virus sauce."

"I didn't plan on us getting a stomach virus."

"So you made cass-oo-let," he said drawing out the syllables.

"Schmuck. You're just saying that to aggravate me."

"I could say that about your menu."

She threw the sheets back to fall crumpled at the foot of the bed. He lay there in his shorts while she was wearing one of his extra large tees and bikini panties. The tee had been laundered into a fine web and the panties had been tight four months ago. Breathing deeply, he unclenched his fingers.

"Good god, what was that?"

"That, twit, was your cooking—the mixing of beans and virus in my gut."

"Don't aim it over here."

"You're not exactly smelling like a flower yourself, Baby Cakes."

"Then turn the other way."

Reaching down, she pulled the sheets up to her neck. He sat up to see her body's impossibly small imprint in the bed. She closed her eyes tightly, scrunching her forehead with the same look of forced detachment he had seen every time the nurses came with the tray of tubes, needles, and bags of fluid. She had been stoic. He was determined to shake her out of the trance.

"Your farts are so potent they could wake the dead. It's why you didn't die isn't it? God was concerned you'd pollute his workplace."

"Not fucking funny. You're just creating a diversion from ... Oh my God that was awful. Should we fumigate?"

Simultaneously, they shoved the sheets off the bed.

"For heaven's sake, don't light a match," he said.

His eyes twinkled with laughter. Her eyes filled with tears.

"Not one of my brightest ideas," she admitted.

"Yeah, but it's the thought that counts. Thanks for making dinner when you didn't feel so good."

"I couldn't stomach toast one more time. And no more casseroles. We needed protein."

"I can give you protein ... "

"Maybe later," she said.

They lay quietly. The morning sun shone through the blinds. The bars of light alternated with unfamiliar shadows of loss.

"Do you miss them?"

"Absolutely but it was no contest. I'd pick you over them any day."

"I miss them too. In the morning, I go to get a bra and then remember."

"We'll buy new ones. Any size you want."

"Do you think it's worth it?"

"It's your body, little skinny one."

She bit her lip. He laid his hand on her shoulder. She quickly shrugged it off. Like she couldn't bear the weight of it. Like she had been doing every time he touched her since the diagnosis.

"Don't know if I want to do more surgery."

"When do you need to make the decision?"

"At some point soon. I've got to go back to work."

"Have you heard from anyone at the office?"

"Some people have called—but apart from sending over those damn casseroles."

"God save us. I never want to see another casserole as long as I live."

"Hmmm. I'd hate to think my last meal would be a casserole."

She patted her body checking to see if she had lost anything else in the night.

"They're still covering for me at work."

"Think you'll be replaced?"

"Not so much that as I want life to go back to normal."

"Normal huh?"

"Well, new normal."

"Do you think the office can stand your GI intrusions, your not so little malodorous gifts?"

"Hey, hey. You know I'm a little touchy."

"In more ways than one."

"No really. Don't tease."

"Sorry. I'm just not sure what topics are off limits."

"Not off limits. More like pause. Could you think before you speak?"

"Ouch that was a little rough."

She looked at where the ceiling and the wall came together. Sniffed. Stiffened her spine. Used her hand to wipe her nose.

"Oh shit. Now I don't know what to say anymore," she said.

"Yeah, well, I feel like I'm walking through a mine field over here."

"It's like there's no safe place. At work, with friends, in our bed."

"Yep. Everything I say is wrong."

"No. Not everything."

She sat up in the bed.

"Do you think the insurance company would pay for new boobs?"

"We can call or better yet have the nurse from the doctor's office call."

"What if they don't?"

"We'll master the moment."

"What if I decide not to reconstruct?"

"Truth?"

"Yes, truth."

"It would take some getting used to. On one hand, you've been through so much. So on most days, I think just being with you is enough. All I can ask for. On the other hand, I like curves."

"I look like a boy?" she said.

"A little. With your hair still so short and being so thin."

"I hate wearing the wig. It hurts but I look like a baby bird – little tufts playing at being hair but mostly I'm just bald."

"It's downy soft. Makes me want to rub it for luck."

"Fuck, fuck, fuck."

"No fuck me," he said. Smiling. Waving his penis at her. Friendly like. He flashed back to the times they would play BC, before cancer. In a high sing song voice, he said, "Hello Ms. Baby Cakes, it's a wonderful day in the neighborhood. Won't you come out and play with my wood?"

"That's funny. Stop it asshole"

"Baby Cakes, you used to think I was funny."

"Now you're making fun of me."

"So what's your point? We used to say you were the lust of my loins, buns to my wiener … "

"Oh. Yeah. Used to say – fucking hilarious. Go ahead. Make a joke out of my cancer."

"Damn right I will. It's been funny at times. You need to face up to it. The gas is funny. The bird look is funny. I love you but it is funny. Not all the time but sometimes."

"I am not funny. Cancer isn't funny. Chemo isn't funny."

"Funny was how we coped from the first date. It's how we'll cope now."

"Don't laugh at me. I can't bear it."

"I have to. We stopped being funny, making jokes, laughing, and things got scary. Then we stopped talking. I miss you."

"But we stayed together. You were there for me. Always."

"Yes, and I don't see me ever not being there for you but we have to lighten up."

"I want the funny back. The jokes and the laughing. But it feels like you are laughing at me, making light of what I went through."

"Hey you set me up. You're the one who makes a frank and beans casserole and then barks at me for making fart jokes."

"Haven't I been through enough?"

"You've been a trooper. And a lot of it you did alone but some of it, we went through together. I wouldn't have had it any other way. I would have done more if you'd let me. I understand you getting sucked in by the medical machinery but you chose it over us."

"You're saying I'm farty from the chemo."

"You didn't hear what I said—you shut me out." He paused to let his words sink in. "And yes you've always been farty. BC, you'd fart in your sleep. It would wake me up but it was somewhat endearing, irritating and smelly but endearing. Then you lost your sense of humor from the chemo. I get that. You still fart. Now it's time to pick it back up – your sense of humor. You said you wanted normal. Well normal for us is being silly, poking fun, having sex."

"I feel tender like my scalp."

"Your hair is growing in. Let your sense of humor grow in too."

He tickled her feet. Along with the giggles came her inevitable toot. He watched her turn pink.

"Whatever possessed you? Beans on a bus."

"Not sure. Maybe wanting to spend some quality time with you. In another city. Not a cancer city."

"Okay but I'm not sitting next to you with this gas. Dangerous to my health."

"Good point," she said wrinkling her nose. "Maybe you can sit at the front of the bus and I'll sit at the back."

"We'll aim our emissions at the middle and smile innocently."

"You are silent but deadly."

"I'm not silent," he said.

"And I'm not dead," she said.

"Yeah, you need to fart like an adolescent boy. All bravado and bullshit."

"Will you stop saying I look like a boy?" she said, cranky, hurt, on the edge of a fight.

"Okay Honey, not a boy so much. Lanky, unsure, like a colt. On second thought, still too much ass for a boy."

"Stop patronizing me."

"We'll do something about the breasts later. The hair and eyebrows are coming back." He searched for the gentler words. "Wear a cap on the bus. We'll confuse them – they'll wonder where all the gas is coming from. To top it off, we'll smooch in all your androgynous beauty."

This time, she let him touch her; caress her in the BC ways. He felt her fight to stay connected to him.

"I'm too sexy for my hair," she sang. He half sighed with relief, half laughed at her first attempt at cancer humor.

"Ain't love grand?" she said.

"And stinky."

"You did that on purpose."

"You bet your fine skinny ass I did."

Beans On A Bus

A diagnosis of breast cancer is not a death sentence. The survival rate has grown to 89.1% at five years post diagnosis with 80% of people diagnosed surviving beyond 10 years. But a diagnosis of breast cancer will change a person's life and the lives of the people around that person. It is estimated that 1 in 8 women will be diagnosed with breast cancer in her lifetime or 5.68% of women will develop breast cancer between the ages of 50 and 70. In 2011, there will be 230,480 women diagnosed with breast cancer in the US and 39,520 women will die of the disease in that year (National Cancer Institute, 2012).

As a woman ages, her chance of developing breast cancer increases. There are eight other major factors increasing the risk of breast cancer for women:

- Inherited genetic changes (Accounts for 10% of breast cancer cases)

- Dense breasts (Making abnormalities more difficult to detect on mammograms)

- Onset of menstruation before age 12 (Breasts appearing earlier in life is correlated with increased risk for breast cancer later in life)

- Onset of menopause after age 55 (Prolonged estrogen production)

- Having a first baby after age 30 (Pregnancy promotes rapid breast cell growth and if there is genetic damage to the breast cells, which tends to increase with age, that will be copied as well)

- Never having been pregnant (Pregnancy and breastfeeding reduce the number of menstrual cycles and a woman's exposure to estrogen)

- Post-menopausal obesity (As a person gains weight, breast tissue can become more fatty. Toxins can bind to the fat in breasts faster than in other organs.)

- Alcohol use (Greater alcohol consumption increases a woman's chance of breast cancer)

A new group of contributing variables is being studied – the environmental pollutants such as the chemical BPA (bisphenol A), pesticides, and second hand smoke. BPA is a ubiquitous plastic additive that mimics estrogen. Exposure can happen on the job, from the use of plastic bottles, and from the linings of food cans. The imitation estrogen, BPA, can lead to obesity with fatter breasts, denser breasts, earlier onset of puberty, and the delay of menopause. Pesticides have been linked to the increased incidence of breast cancer in farmers. Second hand smoke has been linked to increased incidence of breast cancer in workers in bars, casinos, and racetracks.

As of 2010, most breast cancer diagnoses occur in women between the ages of 45 and 54. Diagnosis before age 40 and after the age of 85 is uncommon. It is diagnosed more frequently in White American women but Black American women die more often from the disease.

Breast cancer treatment impacts two major sensitive areas: the sexual activity and the sexual self-esteem of the woman (and man) diagnosed. Treatment includes a combination of some or all of these procedures: surgical removal of lumps, one or both breasts, lymph nodes; complete hysterectomies removing the uterus and both ovaries; chemotherapy; and radiation. The treatments can take up to several years to complete and may continue throughout a woman or man's life. The treatments make changes in the person's body. In women, treatment and surgical protocols can cause a surgical and/or chemical menopause with its resultant changes in body, cognitive ability, sexual activity, and personal identity. Women will have to resolve issues of premature infertility. Many women report feeling shame – they did something to cause this and label themselves as damaged goods. As one woman stated, "How can anyone still feel beautiful and desired after so much has been taken away?"

Many women treated for breast cancer are adamant that the last thing they want is another pair of hands touching them, even loving hands. She may have a premature menopause with vaginal drying making intercourse uncomfortable. Orgasm is different after cancer treatment because sensitivity may be affected by the treatments. There can be a loss of breast stimulation and a decrease in overall body sensation. Surgical removal of the uterus will cause loss of uterine contractions during orgasm. Yeast infections, anal fissures, flare ups of genital warts and herpes along with vaginal and mouth sores may make sex unpleasant, uncomfortable and "not worth the energy," as one woman succinctly stated.

Sex does not need to be stopped during treatment but women and men are cautioned to use a condom for the first few days after a chemotherapy treatment to avoid passing on the chemotherapy drug to their partners. Women having sex with women should use a barrier, such as a dental dam to prevent the transmission of the chemotherapy to her partner.

From diagnosis through treatment and beyond, partners may be confused and distressed. Couples' usual patterns of connection are disrupted. Partners may see their cancer survivor mates as too fragile for sexual activities. People may try to forget the cancer diagnosis and subsequent treatment but it is impossible. Not anyone, be it doctors, nurses, therapists, technicians, patients, their family, friends or partners, will say breast cancer diagnosis and treatment is sexy.

Sexual identity, desire, and functioning for the survivor and her/his partner or partners can be rebuilt. The American Cancer Society has a welcoming and thoughtful website about sexual reconnection. The website suggests women (and men):

- Grieve your losses and changes in your body, mind, spirit, and sexuality. Join a support group or work alone with a trusted friend, clergy or therapist.
- Rewire your sexual responses – sensitivity will be different. You may lack desire from pain, fatigue or bodily changes from the treatment. Get help from a sex therapist (directories can be found in the Resource section). If you are part of a couple, get help together.
- Don't give up – this is an ongoing conversation between the woman and herself and the woman and her partner or partners.
- Be blunt – learn to say what feels good, doesn't feel good or needs a different type of stimulation. Wendy Maltz's book, The Sexual Healing Journey, contains exercises to rebuild trust, open up verbal and nonverbal communication after sexual trauma (breast cancer diagnosis and treatment is sexual trauma).

After treatment's break from the usual pattern of sexual behavior and feelings, the breast cancer survivor will probably have to rebuild her/his sexual self-esteem. The person can read, learn, do exercises alone or with a partner. The survivor can rebuild their connection to their body – take up yoga, meditate, get a massage, learn to give a massage, and exercise (such as kickboxing). These activities have been shown to increase the quality of life of people diagnosed with breast cancer and increase the overall survival rates.

A woman or man must develop a new normal after diagnosis and treatment for breast cancer. Desire can be strengthened. Touch can be relearned as pleasurable and not clinical or painful. Sexuality can be re-established as a form of communication, comfort, and joy.

References:

BioMed Central Limited. "Certain Jobs Linked to Increased Breast Cancer Risk." ScienceDaily, 19 Nov. 2012. Web. 4 Jan. 2013. <http://www.sciencedaily.com/releases/2012/11/121119094512.htm>.

Cancer Statistics Working Group. "US Cancer Statistics 1999-2009 Incidence and Mortality Web-based Report." *Department of Health and Human Services*. CDC, Prevention, National cancer Institute, 20 Mar. 2013. Web. 27 Sept. 2013. <www.cdc.gov/uscs>.

Chustecka, Zosia. "New Guidelines on Chemoprevention for Breast Cancer." *Medscape Multispecialty*. Medscape: Medscape Access, 24 Sept. 2013. Web. 29 Sept. 2013. <http://www.medscape.com/viewarticle/811553>.

Deardorff, Julie. "Facing Post-Treatment Issues: Mapping Out a Care Plan after Treatment Can Help Breast Cancer Survivors Thrive in Body and Mind." *Chicago Tribune News* 26 Sept. 2012: Health. Web. 4 Dec. 2012. <http://articles.chicagotribune.com/2012-09-26/health/sc-health-0926-bc-survivor-20120926_1_breast-cancer-cancer-journey-treatment-ends>.

Gotbaum, Rachel. "Cancer Rehab Begins to Bridge a Gap to Reach Patients." *Shots: Health News from NPR*. NPR, 18 Feb. 2013. Web. 1 Mar. 2013. <http://www.npr.org/blogs/health/2013/02/18/172099043/cancer-rehab-begins-to-bridge-a-gap-to-reach-patients>.

Gubar, Susan. "Living with Cancer: Is It Back?" *New York Times* [New York] 29 Aug. 2013: n. pag. Print.

Howlader, N, A. M. Noone, M. Krapcho, R. Aminou, W. Waldron, S. F. Altekruse, C. L. Kosary, J. Ruhl, Z. Tatalovich, H. Cho, A. Mariotto, M. P. Eisner, H. S. Chen, E. J. Feuer, K. A. Cronin, and B. K. Edwards. "Breast Cancer Risk in American Women." *National Cancer Institute*. National Institute of Health, US Department of Health and Human Services, 24 Sept. 2012. Web. 1 Jan. 2013. <http://www.cancer.gov/cancertopics/factsheet/detection/probability-breast-cancer>.

Jennings, Dana. "Losing a Comforting Ritual: Treatment." *The New York Times* 29 June 2009: n. pag. Web. 4 Dec. 2012. <http://www.nytimes.com/2009/06/30/health/30case.html?_r=0>.

Maticka-Tyndale, University of Windsor. "New Study Targets High-Risk Occupations for Breast Cancer." University of Windsor, 19 Nov. 2012. Web. 4 Jan. 2013. <http://www.uwindsor.ca/dailynews/2012-11-18/new-study-targets-high-risk-occupations-for-breast-cancer>.

Surveillance Epidemiology and End Results. "SEER Stat Fact Sheets: Breast cancer." *National Cancer Institute*. National Institutes of Health, US Department of Health and Human Services, Apr. 2013. Web. 26 Sept. 2013. <http://seer.cancer.gov/statfacts/html/breast.html>.

www.cancer.org (website of the American Cancer Society)

Activity 1

Keep a Sexual Desire Diary. For two weeks, every time you have a sexual thought or feeling write it down. Note:

Date and time

Alone or with some one

What you did with the thought or feeling (did you ignore the thought/feeling, save it for later or act on it then)

How would you have liked to have acted on the thought or feeling?

After two weeks, see if any patterns emerge. Use the information to explore and strengthen your sexuality.

Activity 2

To relearn touch, use Wendy Maltz's guidelines of three important skills (Maltz, p. 252).

1). Relax and rest (take a break when you notice your breathing has become erratic or uncomfortable).

2). Practice active awareness (stop when you check out, become numb, or uncomfortable).

3). Be creative in your problem solving when you hit a snag physically or emotionally (adapt activities and exercises to your personal needs).

This two-part exercise will slow down your usual pattern of sexual behaviors and allow for new behaviors to develop. Do this with your doctor's permission. Do the first part of the exercise alone. When you are comfortable with the first part of the activity and if you have a partner, practice the second part of the activity. Remember to take as much time as you need (over days and months), stop when you are overwhelmed or checked out and modify the exercises to fit your body and needs (using Maltz's three guidelines).

Part 1: By yourself and over as much time (days or months) as you need:

Start by wrapping your arms around the breast area and breathe (first contact with your body).

Then put your hands over the breasts or breast area and firmly hold them.

Increase the pressure and start to gently rock them (feel the sensations over the skin and bones of the area).

Run a wet towel around your breasts and breast area (try cold, lukewarm, and almost hot towels)

Smooth on some oil or lotion (nothing abrasive or exfoliating).

Massage your breast area (notice the differences in sensation with different strokes, pressure, parts of your hands).

Find methods of touching your breasts and breast area that bring on sexual pleasure.

Find a way to document how it is in your body to have breasts (with words, collages, photos, recordings, videos).

What did you like about Part 1? Not like? Why? Did certain images or memories come up? Is there something you would like to change from this process?

Part 2: With a partner, after having established the three guidelines above and over as much time (days or months) as you need:

Have your partner wrap their arms around you in a close hug. Feel their breast area next to your breast area and breathe (first contact between you and your partner).

Then have your partner put their hands over your breasts or breast area and firmly hold the breasts/the breast area.

Have the partner increase the pressure and start to gently rock the breasts or breast area (feel the sensations over the skin and bones of the area).

Have your partner run a wet towel around your breasts and breast area (try cold, lukewarm, and almost hot towels).

Have your partner smooth on some oil or lotion (nothing abrasive or exfoliating).

Have your partner massage your breast area (notice the differences in sensation with different strokes, pressure, parts of their hands).

Encourage your partner to find methods of touching your breasts and breast area that bring on sexual pleasure.

Find a way to document how it is in your body to have breasts in contact with another breast area (with words, collages, photos, recordings, videos). What did you like in Part 2? Not like? Why? Did certain images or memories come up? Is there something you would like to change from this process?

Talk, if you like, to your partner about the process. What were their responses? What did they like? Not like? What came up for them in the form of images, memories, and feelings? Is there something they would like to change from this exercise?

Activity 3

Within a group, brainstorm aloud.

How are breasts connected to femininity? And masculinity?

How are breasts connected to sexuality? Is the connection to sexuality different for women and men?

How do you respond if a partner does not like their breasts/breast area being touched?

How would you tell a partner not to touch your breasts?

How would sex change for you if you couldn't have your breasts/breast area touched?

How would sex change for you if you couldn't touch your partner's breasts/breast area?

Why do you think some women choose not to go through surgical reconstruction of their breasts?

If having the lights on feels too daunting, turn off the lights, put a candle in the middle of the room and add some soft music in the background (try New Age instrumentals that can change the breathing patterns to a more even and relaxed pattern). With this little bit of anonymity and camouflage, the exercise can become easier and less embarrassing.

Resources:

American Cancer Society at www.cancer.org has helpful sections on "Rekindling Sexuality"

Brooks, Linda, and Jacques Brisson. "Medscape: Medscape Access." *Do Breast Implants Affect Breast Cancer Survival? An Expert Interview with Jacques Brisson, MD, DSc*. Medscape Internal Medicine, 17 July 2013. Web. 26 Oct. 2013. <http://www.medscape.com/viewarticle/807776>.

Maltz, Wendy. *The Sexual Healing Journey: A Guide for Survivors of Sexual Abuse*. New York, NY: HarperPerrenial, 1991. Print. (While this is a book for survivors of sexual abuse, it contains a series of exercises to rebuild comfort in touch and teach communication for sexual partners.)

Living Beyond Breast Cancer. N.p., n.d. Web. 27 Nov. 2013. <http://www.lbbc.org/>.

"Not Just Surviving - Thriving! Life Beyond Breast Cancer ... " *Tough Warrior Princesses*. N.p., n.d. Web. 27 Nov. 2013. <http://survivethenthrive.blogspot.com/>.

Shaw, Gina. "Breast Caner Survivors: Life after the Treatment Ends. The Breast Cancer Treatments are Over. Now What? Here's How to Return to Your "New Normal."." *Breast Cancer Health Center.* WedMD, 2005. Web. 4 Dec. 2012. <http://www.webmd.com/breast-cancer/guide/life-after-breast-cancer-treatment>.

Directories of sex therapists include:

American Association of Couples and Sex Therapists (www.aacast.net)

American Association of Sex Educators, Counselors and Therapists (www.aasect.org)

Society for Sex Therapy and Research (www.sstarnet.org)

Lord Almighty

"Lord Almighty, she's going to cut off her breasts," Shirley wailed into the phone holding her daughter's baby picture with the other hand. Tears ran down Shirley's face. Her nose was swollen to the point she had to stretch her mouth wide to take in a breath. "I tell you. I don't know what's going on. We thought Jeanie was trying to get some attention. Shock us. She'd lose her nerve but the surgery's happening as we speak."

Shirley stared at her white knuckles ending in the red fingers of tense imaginings. The growing silence on the telephone line forced Shirley to tune back in. "Yes, I know she's supposed to have had two years counseling but she hooked up with some quack doctor near the school."

A pink roly-poly baby smiled up at her from the Polaroid. "She was such a beautiful little girl. I don't understand. What would make her do this?" There was some more babbling from the phone friend.

"I don't know. I just don't know. She went back to college sad, withdrawn after the break up with Ronnie. We didn't hear from her for a while. She didn't return our phone calls. I even drove out there one weekend to say hi. Did I handle this wrong?" The phone mumbled.

Shirley stared at the collection of family photo albums neatly stacked on the coffee table. "If there was a way for me to have stopped this I would have. But she's twenty-one, legally an adult. The attorney said there was nothing we could do."

Shirley concentrated hard on the phone. The lines on her face catching more tears. "Of course we contacted the school. Now Jeanie won't talk to us. According to her, if we don't support this surgery, we're against her. She claims it's not a snap decision. Of course, we're against this surgery. No reasonable woman would cut off her breasts."

Shirley sat on the couch with the cordless phone. A dog came over and laid its head on her lap. "The school was no help. The counselor gave me a list of resources to help me understand the process," she snipped off each word waving her daughter's picture fast and furious. "I don't want to understand the process." The baby girl fluttered out of her hand, twirled in the air to land on top of the coffee table's albums.

"She wants us to call her Jim now. Jeanie, Jennette, Jean makes her scream. My therapist says it's the testosterone and the need to establish a new identity. I think Dr. Little was as distressed as I was. She kept babbling on about the need for therapy, like we would refuse to pay to stop this mutilation. I begged Jeanie to go to therapy but I can't make her go. The school can't make her go. Do you think it's just a reaction to the break up with her boyfriend? What did we do wrong?"

The screen door slammed shut. Shirley jumped. The dog rolled her eyes upward but refused to move its head from her lap. Her husband walked in. "Have you heard anything?" Shirley asked covering the phone with her hands. Dave looked back blankly.

"What. About what?" he said.

"Dave, it's about Jeanie. The surgery. Has she called you?"

"No, you're her mother. She would have called you. Did she call?" His blood shot gaze traveled the room to focus on his steel-toed boots. Face hidden by more than his five o'clock shadow.

"What?" Shirley's voice escalated to the sound right before yelling.

"Don't raise your voice at me," he snarled. His voice boomed through the house. "This is your fault. She's your daughter."

"What are you talking about? It's our baby girl." Shirley reached out to her husband with one hand while holding the phone in her other hand.

"Get off the phone. Get off the damn phone." His breathing was harsh and fast.

"I got to go," and Shirley put the cordless phone into the cradle of its charger. "Dave, we got to do something."

"You should have thought of that before now," he said looking at her with hard, accusing eyes.

"I tried everything I could think of. The attorney, her pediatrician, her therapist, my therapist, the counselor at school, even the doctor prescribing the meds. I can't get the name of the surgeon. I don't even know where our daughter is. She's not thinking right."

"You should have done more." Clenched fists at the sides of a blocky torso strained the buttons of his checkered shirt.

"You're accusing me. What more was there I could do? Why didn't you do something? All this time, you made me the bad parent. You empathized and listened. You turned Jeanie against me. You turned her against being a woman." The veins in Shirley's neck pulsed.

Dave continued to stare at his wife. The contempt flattening his mouth as he loomed over her.

"Why don't you say it? Why don't you say you hate me? You blame me for everything," Shirley was full out screaming now. The tears and runny nose mixing on her face, dripping down to stain her blouse.

Dave stood over her. "I don't hate you," he said speaking every last word with the same thunderous tone. He collapsed stone-heavy on the edge of the couch. Their dog lurched out of Shirley's lap to squeeze its body between them. The dog sat upright, a canine buffer between two opponents. The couple looked at each other with twenty-four years of hushed-up resentment. Ten beats passed.

Shirley watched Dave's body deflate. The features of his face shrank, cheeks hollowing, eyes receding. His arms hugged his chest. Heavy thighs spread lax. Dave's entire being rocked, defeated.

"I don't understand you," he said through his own tears.

Shirley absently moved over to give the dog more room. "It's my baby girl. I couldn't stop this. You couldn't stop this."

He repeated, "I don't understand her or you."

Shirley looked at him, seeing for the first time how he had aged from the young buck she fell in love with into a despairing middle-aged man. "I want my baby back," she said, unsure whether she was talking about her daughter, her husband, or both. Shirley gently moved the dog off the couch to close the gap between them. She laid a tentative arm around her husband's shoulders. The dog lay on the floor wedged between the couple and the coffee table—its velvety ears flopped over their feet like a living comforter. Dave stopped the rocking of his body. Shirley smoothed the familiar ruffle of hair on his head. A low wail escaped him and Shirley's hand guided Dave's head onto her chest.

Lord Almighty

Most people confuse the definitions of sex and gender. Sex is the biological state of an animal or human being determined by chromosomes and anatomical structures. Gender is determined by culture (sex, social roles, and gender identity). Gender identity is the classification that the person self-identifies with. The US Caucasian society recognizes two sexes (female and male) and two genders (male and female). Many societies recognize more than two genders. Different North American tribes have recognized more than two genders with the other gender classifications labeled as shamans and healing individuals. Prior to the 19th century, the Incas, Egyptians, Italians, and some tribes in Siberia recognized more than two genders. Indigenous peoples in Hawaii, Indonesia, the Philippines, New Zealand, and the Dominican Republic recognize at least four different genders. Today, Tamil recognizes 20 different genders. U.S. Psychology and counseling programs consider androgynous characteristics (not exclusively female or male) preferable for their health care professionals.

Transgendered people have a gender identity that is different from the biological state they were born with or assigned at birth when biological anatomy is unclear. They are estimated to make up between 0.0025% and 1% of the general US population. Transgendered people are biological males changing or changed to female and biological females changing or changed to male by the processes of behavioral expression, hormonal therapy, sexual reassignment surgery, and cosmetic surgery.

Surgery is considered the third and final stage of the change. Seventy-six percent of people who undergo surgery to change from male to female are happy with the results. Breast removal is the most common surgery requested by women transitioning to men. Breast removal is considered a cosmetic surgery but is not considered a genital surgery. Many women changing to men elect to have their breasts removed early in the transformation process. "Top surgery," as it is called, is a double mastectomy with chest contouring and nipple repositioning to shape a more masculine appearing chest. As not all breast tissue is removed, it is important to have continuous screening for breast cancer and diseases. Thailand performs the most sex reassignment surgeries in the world followed by Iran.

Transgendered individuals in the US face violence, discrimination, and fear. November 20th is Transgender Day of Remembrance where victims of violence against transgendered individuals are commemorated. From 1998 to November of 2011, 320 transgendered people died from hate crimes in the US. A horrific example occurred on August 26, 2011 when an off-duty 20-year veteran of the Washington, D.C. police force stood on the hood of a car and shot through the windshield at the two transgendered women and their male friend sitting in their car.

For the first time in US history, in 2009, President Obama included violence against transgendered people in the legal category of hate crimes. In a poll of 6500 transgendered Americans, 26% report some form of violence or physical assault because they are transgendered and half of the polled individuals are wary of asking for police assistance. Fifty percent of all lethal anti-LGBT (lesbian, gay, bisexual, transgendered) hate crimes are committed against transgendered women and girls. Sexual assault is being recognized as a serious problem for the transgender population. Most transgendered people in the US report being sexually assaulted in some form.

Forms of discrimination reported include being incarcerated, evicted or fired along with being ostracized, harassed, and ridiculed. The average annual income for a transgendered individual is reported at less than $10,000 – transgendered individuals are between four and five time more likely to live in extreme poverty than the general population – despite 85% of transgendered individuals finishing some college versus the national average of 57 percent.

This sexualization and marginalization by the media has made created a climate contributing to the high rate of sexual assault of transgendered individuals. The media portrays transgendered people as hookers, cocaine addicts, and prostitutes. A survey by the National Center for Transgender Equality found 41% of respondents had attempted suicide.

References:

Ahmed, Beenish. "Violent Attacks on Transgender People Raise Alarm." *News - U.S. - Law: Morning Edition*. NPR, 29 Sept. 2011. Web. 26 Jan. 2013. <http://www.npr.org/2011/09/29/140877153/violent-attacks-on-transgender-people-raise-alarm>.

AETNA. "Clinical Policy Bulletin: Gender Reassignment Surgery." *AETNA*. AETNA Inc., 15 Oct. 2013. Web. 18 Nov. 2013. <http://www.aetna.com/cpb/medical/data/600_699/0615.html>.

"Community Conversation: Insurance Coverage." *Transgender Resources*. Susan's Place, 20 May 2011. Web. 21 Jan. 2013. <http://www.susans.org/forums/index.php?topic=98784.0>.

Empire Blue. "Gender Reassignment Surgery." *Clinical UM Guideline*. Empire HealthChoice Assurance, 8 Aug. 2013. Web. 29 Oct. 2013. <http://www.empireblue.com/medicalpolicies/guidelines/gl_pw_a051166.htm>.

"Ending Anti-Transgender Violence." *NCTE Blueprint for Equality 2012*. National Center for Transgender Equality, 2012. Web. 26 Jan. 2013. <http://transequality.org/Resources/NCTE_Blueprint_for_Equality2012_Ending_Violence.pdf>.

Enfield, Michelle. "Transgender Woman Learns to Embrace Uniqueness." *News - Opinion - Commentary.* NPR, n.d. Web. 26 Jan. 2013. <http://www.npr.org/2011/06/23/137369283/transgender-woman-learns-to-embrace-uniqueness>.

Grant, Jaime M., Lisa A. Mottet, Justin Tanis, Jack Harrison, Jody L. Herman, and Mara Keisling. "Injustice at Every Turn: A Report of the National Transgender Discrimination Survey." *The Task Force.* National Center for Transgender Equality, National Gay and Lesbian Task Force, 2011. Web. 29 Oct. 2011. <http://www.thetaskforce.org/downloads/reports/reports/ntds_summary.pdf>.

Martin, Michelle. "Study: Discrimination Takes a Toll on Transgender Americans." *News - U.S: Tell Me More.* NPR, 28 Mar. 2011. Web. 26 Jan. 2013. <http://www.npr.org/2011/03/28/134926352/Study-Discrimination-Takes-A-Toll-On-Transgendered-Americans>.

Maza, Carlos. "Fox Hosts Mock, Laugh at Transgender Inmate's Appearance." *Media Matters.* Media Matters for America, 11 Jan. 2013. Web. 18 Jan. 2013.

NCTE. "Understanding Transgender." *Frequently Asked questions About Transgender People*. National center for Transgender Equality, May 2009. Web. 26 Jan. 2013. <http://transequality.org/Resources/NCTE_UnderstandingTrans.pdf>.

"Sex Reassignment Surgery." *Wikipedia: The Free Encyclopedia*. Wikimedia Foundation, Inc., 2013. Web. 29 Oct. 2013. <http://en.wikipedia.org/wiki/Sex_reassignment_surgery>.

"Sex Reassignment Therapy." *Wikipedia: The Free Encyclopedia*. Wikimedia Foundation, Inc., 2013. Web. 29 Oct. 2013. <http://en.wikipedia.org/wiki/Sex_reassignment_therapy>.

Transgender at Work. "Transgender Health Benefits." Transgender At Work, Web. 29 Oct. 2013. <http://www.tgender.net/taw/tsins.html>.

"Transgender Issues: A Fact Sheet." Transgenderlaw.org, Web. 21 Jan. 2013. <http://www.transgenderlaw.org/resources/transfactsheet.pdf>.

"Transgender Surgery." *Transgendered Explored*. Transgenderexplored, n.d. Web. 21 Jan. 2013.

"Transition and Insurance." *Transsexual Road Map*. GenderLife, 6 Mar. 2013. Web. 29 Oct. 2013. <http://www.tsroadmap.com/reality/insurance.html>.

Activity 1

Make six columns.

In the first column list all the words associated with female. Draw a symbol for this group.

Summarize the themes or common ideas associated with each group of words. Are they positive, negative, or neutral?

In the second column list all the words associated with male. Draw a symbol for this group.

Summarize the themes or common ideas associated with each group of words.

Are they positive, negative, or neutral?

In the third column list all the words associated with biological females transitioning to male. Draw a symbol for this group.

Summarize the themes or common ideas associated with each group of words.

Are they positive, negative, or neutral?

In the fourth column list all the words associated with biological males transitioning to female. Draw a symbol for this group.

Summarize the themes or common ideas associated with each group of words.

Are they positive, negative, or neutral?

In the fifth column list all the words associated with androgynous people. Draw a symbol for this group.

Summarize the themes or common ideas associated with each group of words.

Are they positive, negative, or neutral?

In the sixth column list all the words associated with asexual people. Draw a symbol for this group.

Summarize the themes or common ideas associated with each group of words.

Are they positive, negative, or neutral?

What group of words is more comfortable for you? Do you know why?

Activity 2

What jobs and activities are gender-specific? How could they become available to different sexes and genders? Why are they segregated?

What is your policy on transgendered athletes, teachers, prison guards, and medical providers? Should the people they represent or give care to be told? Who should tell them?

Activity 3

Watch the video segment on Bill O'Reilly and Megyn Kelly dated 01/11/2013 discussing the use of taxpayer monies to help prisoners with the surgeries for transition to male to female. (http://mediamatters.org/blog/2013/01/11/fox-hosts-laugh-at-transgender-inmates-app/1912191)

Should taxpayer monies be used this way?

What is the rationale for using monies for these surgeries?

What did you think about O'Reilly's statement about the transgendered male to female prisoner being unattractive?

Should a male to female transgendered prisoner be incarcerated in a male prison?

What constitutes beauty or attractiveness?

Resources:

AETNA. "Clinical Policy Bulletin: Gender Reassignment
  Surgery." *AETNA*. AETNA Inc., 15 Oct. 2013. Web.
  18 Nov. 2013. <http://www.aetna.com/cpb/medical/
  data/600_699/0615.html>.

"Community Conversation: Insurance Coverage."
  Transgender Resources. Susan's Place, 20 May 2011.
  Web. 21 Jan. 2013. <http://www.susans.org/forums/
  index.php?topic=98784.0>.

NCTE. "Understanding Transgender." *Frequently Asked
  questions About Transgender People*. National
  center for Transgender Equality, May 2009. Web.
  26 Jan. 2013. <http://transequality.org/Resources/
  NCTE_UnderstandingTrans.pdf>.

Transgender at Work. "Transgender Health Benefits."
  Transgender At Work, Web. 29 Oct. 2013. <http://
  www.tgender.net/taw/tsins.html>.

"Transgender Issues: A Fact Sheet." Transgenderlaw.org,
  Web. 21 Jan. 2013. <http://www.transgenderlaw.org/
  resources/transfactsheet.pdf>.

"Transgender Surgery." *Transgendered Explored*.

Transgenderexplored, n.d. Web. 21 Jan. 2013.

"Transition and Insurance." *Transsexual Road Map*. GenderLife, 6 Mar. 2013. Web. 29 Oct. 2013. <http://www.tsroadmap.com/reality/insurance.html>.

Malignancy

Jeffrey was sitting in his office almost panting, feet heavy in his shoes and clothes sticky on his body. His long tapered fingers held a framed picture of himself from college – healthy and trim in Speedos with water beading on his pore-less brown skin. In the photograph's background, his brother Daniel, the only person who knew about his fear of heights, was cheering after Jeffrey's last collegiate dive, a two and a half somersaulting pike barely making a splash on entry. Daniel had been his rock. At every competition. Talking him out of his terror in the locker room and the last person Jeffrey looked at before the dizzying climb up the diving platform. Each dive had been a breath-stealing act of survival quietly recognized by his brother. But today the picture did not comfort or reassure. Sweat rolled down his face to form a puddle on the forty-year old picture. The stink of decay and betrayal tainted the air in the room. *If he could see me now*, Jeffrey was sure his brother would snatch away his medals, his scholarships, and break the picture.

In the last few months, his life had gotten away from him. His department and the conference had moved beyond his control. He had turned away from the lifelines, his wife, a few colleagues and friends, his work. His own body had abandoned him. A furious sense of impotence choked his body making his movements clumsy and his decisions unsure.

The decline began as a slight hesitation like the initial whiff of chlorine rising from a pool. He had found a slight puckering under his nipple. Just a crinkling under the skin about a half-inch long that had not been there the last time he looked at his chest in the mirror. Jeffrey pushed it out of his mind for a month before mentioning the curiosity at his routine blood pressure appointment.

"Probably benign, just a fatty tumor or a cyst," the doctor had said after running a gloved hand over the mass.

"Sure."

"Your blood pressure's still a little high. Think about getting some more exercise. Maybe running. You used to run. Maybe a yoga class. Doesn't your wife do yoga? It would help with the weight and the blood pressure."

Jeffrey had flashed back to his wife saying she felt conspicuous being the only black face in a sea of skinny white girls wearing neon spandex. Jeffrey had pulled all the emotion out of his face. *Black men don't do yoga. Not happening.* But he had said, "Sure. I'll think about it."

Jeffrey had not been amused by the doctor's statement nor had he been comforted. *You try running a department. You find time to exercise. And the last thing I'm gonna do is put on some spandex to touch my toes*, thought Jeffrey.

The doctor had left the room then a minute later knocked and popped his head through the door looking perplexed. He asked Jeffrey to finish getting dressed and come back to his office. Jeffrey was irritated by the lengthy visit but like an obedient child had buttoned his shirt, fixed his tie, and picked up his jacket to follow the signs to the doctor's office. Upon entering, the doctor had looked up from his charts to fix his face into a compassionate smile. Jeffrey felt his foot slipping as he climbed the diving ladder.

"Looking at your family history. Don't you have a brother who had breast cancer?"

"Yes. But it was taken care of. A couple of years ago. Daniel hasn't said anything else about it."

"Well we should make certain there's nothing else to this. Just a precaution."

"What?"

"We should follow this up."

All the blood had rushed to Jeffrey's head. "You think I have cancer? Breast cancer?"

"I think we should be prudent. Did they check to see if your brother carried the genes? BRCA 1 or 2?"

The doctor had pronounced it BRACK-AH and Jeffrey was uncertain what letters were included in the designation.

"I didn't hear anything about it. He had surgery. Some radiation. He said it was nothing really."

"Okay well I'm going to send you to a breast specialist. She's good and will check up on this."

"Really? Now? Work's heating up. The department's

putting on a conference."

"Jeffrey, you have some risk factors – your race, the weight gain, the position of the lump. These masses are typically benign but it's important to determine what it is. She'll probably just run some tests and send you home with a clean bill of health."

Jeffrey had felt the gorge rise up, scramble his heartbeat, and stiffen his breath. He looked at the smooth surface of the water shimmering crystal hard, surrounded by the dull gray of cement and knew himself to be alone.

When the office of the breast specialist called to confirm the appointment, he had said, "Sure, I'll be there." But as the day of the appointment approached, he waivered. Several times, he picked up the phone to cancel the visit. He told no one about "the useless waste of my time" as he called it.

Dutifully, he had turned up at the appointment ten minutes early to "fill out forms." The specialist was forty-five minutes late. He fumed. With barely a hello, Jeffrey was being felt up by a doctor, a white female doctor at that, poking and prodding his chest. Unexpectedly, her fingers had fumbled. The doctor said with a casual delivery, "It's good you came. It's important we check these things out early … " Then, she thumped on his abdomen, watched the jiggle, and thumped again. "Let's see how healthy you are."

Jeffrey snorted.

The doctor sent him to the room next door. A lab technician cuffed his arm and snapped the protective cover off a long needle. The tech looked bored as she drained tube after tube of blood from his body before plastering the puncture with a pink flowered bandage explaining, "Breast cancer awareness month." Jeffrey wondered who had picked October. He was hustled back to wait in the exam room.

Jeffrey had sat alone, staring at the pictures of women in affirming poses and some god-awful poster of a woman with a tattoo where her breast should have been. The room was cold. Jeffrey shivered in the pastel paper gown, his underwear and socks. Looking around, he grabbed a blanket from a pile on the counter and tried to wrap the delicately crocheted material around his waist. The fabric caught on the metal stirrups sticking out from under the table. He jerked at the blanket. The weave held and the stirrups pulled all the way out with a loud scraping noise. Jeffrey tore the blanket free of the metal footholds as he tried to imagine how a man could feel at ease in a room with those stirrups, especially a pink ruffled room. The pastel paper gown stuck to his underarms as he waited. Should he get dressed now?

Just as he stood up, the doctor came back into the room. Like a good patient, he sat back down on the table. With a nod, she had turned her back to him, making notes in the chart and had started asking questions in a flat but vigilant manner.

"How much do you drink? Each night?"

"Not much."

"Every night?"

"A scotch when I get home."

"On a big night?"

"I'm not much of a drinker." Inwardly Jeffrey called her an impertinent ball buster.

"Do you know you have an enlarged liver?"

"What? How would I know?"

The doctor had pushed the stirrups back into the hidden slots under the table. Jeffrey jumped at the noise.

"Enlarged livers can be a symptom of male breast cancer. I want you to have some tests." She said something about a sequence of surgery and genetic profiling.

"You're not going to do a mammogram?" Jeffrey asked.

"No need. While some men have mammograms, your mass is palpable. We'll just proceed to the next step."

"What's the next step?"

"I'll aspirate a little bit of the tissue and check for cancer cells."

"When are you going to do that?"

"Right now."

"Huh?" Jeffrey was spinning from the speed of the

process.

"Yes. Get it over with today and then some blood tests for genetic markers. Just to be safe. Do you have daughters?"

"Yes. Why do you ask?"

"Well. If something turns up, we need to know for your daughters. You could pass on the genes."

The doctor numbed the area with a stinging injection. Smiling blandly at him, she inserted a fine needle into the mass. Jeffrey had not felt a thing.

"All done," she said.

Jeffrey looked down to see a tiny speck of blood. He glared at the nurse offering him another pink bandage. Then the doctor slapped a lab order at him. Jeffrey's hand shook as he took the order from her. He saw she had checked the boxes for BRCA1 and 2 genetic testing.

"Do you need something for anxiety?"

Shocked by the suggestion, Jeffrey said, "Of course not."

"You can get dressed now. Someone from my office will phone you with the results. In a week." The doctor offered a limp fish handshake and left.

For a good ten minutes, Jeffrey had sat in the exam room before he had enough breath to get dressed. He had balled up the pink paper gown and thrown it away. Then he picked it back up from its place next to a basket of sanitary pads, tampons, and tissues. Methodically, beginning at the seams, he ripped the plastic backed paper into five segments. Each segment was shredded into ten pieces before being balled up and thrown into the trash.

Leaving the office, the doctor's Superbill had taunted Jeffrey from the private breast pocket of his jacket. The full-page form was scribbled with procedures and diagnosis in damning medical jargon. *The sheet is pink, that horrific shade of Pepto Bismal pink, another reminder of that miserable female disease*, he thought.

He had been on edge all week. Every corner he turned threatened vertigo. The smell of dead fish drying in the sun assaulted him whenever he opened a book. Students didn't come for office hours - fearful of his bad mood. Colleagues jumped when he entered a room and stopped talking. His co-chair for the conference broke protocol to ask him if things were okay at home. He looked at the woman, plain but attractive in that WASP old money way, and wanted to slap her. The days sped up and slowed down. He felt the diving board's rough surface scraping his feet as he moved his toes to grip the very edge. The water seemed a long way down.

He had been at home when the call came. After five days of being unable to focus, finally he was able to work on grading exams. Papers were spread out on the table. His wife came upon him crying in his chair, head down, shoulders rounded. The needle biopsy had found something and he was to have outpatient surgery, a lumpectomy. They would slice him open. Jeffrey was repulsed by his own smell – panic mixed with disgust. *A fucking woman's disease. Goddamn his brother.* His body was covered in a cold slime of fright. His shirt reeked. He told his wife she would have to drive him to an appointment.

"What do mean?" she said.

"I am having a lumpectomy. I need you to drive me to the hospital."

"What? A lumpectomy? Like for breast cancer?"

"You heard me. A lumpectomy. Can you get off work?"

"Sure Jeff. But what is this all about?"

She had looked so sad. Then she got angry.

"Why didn't you tell me about this?"

He came close to yelling but held his breath. He looked into the dark unforgiving water.

"I don't want to talk about it."

She had walked out of room but on the appointed date had driven him to the outpatient surgery check-in. He told her to wait in the lobby. He would do this alone. Her face crumbled as she drove off to park the car. Luckily, the hospital was sterile lacking the silly posters full of vapid positivity. *You can't make it to department head if you live by those sappy clichés*, he thought turning the words into a mantra pushing the terror into a faraway corner. After the procedure he waived off the radiology technician's concern saying he could dress himself. As she walked out, he felt a threatening wobble of the diving board. He sniffed the rank wet cotton of his shirt.

Against medical orders to rest for a few days, Jeffrey insisted his wife drive him to work. Back in his campus office, he had thrown the undershirt in the trash and re-buttoned his shirt over the three inch long wound. Colleagues had noticed the band-aid showing through the heavily starched and pristine expanse of Jeffrey's shirt. He brushed off their inquiries and offers of help. He called his wife to pick him up.

Between the doctors' appointments and the endless wait for results, Jeffrey had let the ball drop on planning the conference. Alone in his office, he would find himself staring at his diving photograph, mentally rehearsing each dive, and searching for the feeling of controlled flight before the piercing entry into water. When his mind snapped back to the present, he would find his hand hovering over the phone. *I must call Daniel. He'll know what to do.* Daniel could always calm him before a dive.

Jeffrey never made the call. He had so little control remaining. His colleagues' ability to carry on without him made him humorless and hyper-vigilant. He felt himself wobble into a free-fall as the water rushed up to smack him.

He had lost control of the dive's entry. While the

pathologist reported clean margins from the lumpectomy, the tumor's cells were hormone receptor positive. In a mad rush, he was scheduled for a course of radiation to start in three weeks followed by five years of hormone therapy. *Male fucking menopause.* He wasn't asked about his treatment preferences. He was told. He was just another patient in the pipeline.

Jeffrey seethed as he sent out a memo changing his office hours but outlining his expectations to be included in all planning meetings for the upcoming conference.

"So why the change?" asked a colleague.

"Nothing much. Following up on a personal issue. Nothing that will impact my work."

"Well. I'm here if you want to talk about it."

She had smiled kindly at him.

"No need," he had said but the need to tell someone overcame his usual reticence. "I'm having radiation. In the mornings for the next six weeks. They've cut it out – a little growth. Nothing to worry about."

"So sorry to hear this."

"Don't make a big thing out of it."

Jeffrey had brushed off the offer but he felt tainted by the admission. Somehow less powerful. Human and vulnerable. He didn't sleep that night or the next, right up to the night of the surgery. Recovery was more painful than he expected from the surgical literature and consultations.

Moving his arms hurt. Breathing deeply hurt. He changed his order at the cleaners to starch in the cuffs and collar only. Over the next three weeks, the pain abated.

Maybe this is tolerable, he thought. He spent time at work and started to sleep at night with the medications.

When he had begun radiation, Jeffrey felt as if he had hit the water belly first. Lungs popping from the impact of the bad entry. The internal bruising was more painful than he let on. The medical machine gobbled up his dignity and accomplishments with its demand for daily treatment appointments and the dark promise of side effects. When he got a few minutes with his oncologist after the first week of radiation, he had tried to convince the doctor that he didn't need the whole treatment. The technician in the room looked away. The doctor shook his head.

"This is the protocol. It works."

"Why do I need the whole six weeks? I feel fine."

"You want to be around to see your children get married don't you?"

Jeffrey seethed. The oncologist picked up his chart to leave. Jeffrey tried appealing to him man to man.

"I'm having some of the side effects we talked about."

The oncologist asked about the side effects, noted them in the chart, but told Jeffrey to continue the treatment regimen.

"That's not unexpected. Give yourself some time," said

the oncologist.

"I don't have time. I have a department to run and my wife is worrying. This isn't good for her."

"We can get her hooked up with a support group."

"I'm sure they'll have fun. All doing yoga together."

"Jeffrey. It's normal to be scared. There are support groups for you too. But not following the treatment could leave your wife a widow prematurely. Is that what you want?"

"No."

Jeffrey had breathed deep into his chest to stop himself from grabbing the chart from the doctor and ripping up page after page of lies. Or hitting the doctor with it. The doctor beamed a wide smile at him.

"This is the best treatment regimen. Along with hope," the doctor said. "Always look on the bright side."

After the oncologist had left, Jeffrey's body shook with anger. The technician had difficulty positioning his tightly bound body. The appointment took longer than expected and his wife sent word through a bored Candy Striper – asking if he was okay. Jeffrey looked away. He was in no mood to respond. The technician whispered some words and hustled her out of the room.

His wife had sat patiently beside him in the radiology waiting room for each visit. Sometimes she would hand over magazine articles with inspirational stories while his mind whirled with issues of impotence and hot flashes and death. Last week, he had knocked the magazine out of her hands. She started to cry and the other women glared at him. One woman had looked at him with pity as she walked across the room with a tissue box for his wife.

What about me, he had wanted to say. *What if I don't care about nipple sensation and breast reconstruction? What if I can't get it up? What if I have to wear a diaper? What if they have to cut out my balls? How many more ways can you take away my manhood?* But the whole experience was tailored to women. Women technicians. Pink robes. Pictures of women. Even the choice of magazines was female – Vogue, Home and Garden, and the ever-present Breast Cancer Wellness Magazine with its smiling pictures of white women on the front and large hot pink lettering. *Damned if I'm going to read that.* Jeffrey had never felt as disenfranchised as sitting in that waiting room.

As the days and treatments wore on, Jeffrey's tiredness morphed into exhaustion. Rest did not help. Naps did not help. The skin of his chest peeled and formed wet blisters. Again, he changed his order at the dry cleaners. No starch anywhere. His wife had reached out to the support group to find him the softest of undershirts. He was grateful but could not come to say thank you.

During his last week of radiation, when even walking to his office took all his effort, his department members had filed into his office with a gaily-wrapped box. Jeffrey sat up as straight as he could muster. They had bought him a pink tie. Initially, Jeffrey laughed and tied it around his neck.

"Why did you get me a pink tie?"

"To show support and all."

"Support for what?"

"Well we didn't think you'd want a pink ribbon."

"Oh very funny."

Jeffrey patted the tie, thanked them again but was horrified. When they left the office, he took off the tie and wadded it into a ball before hurling it into the trash. A minute later, he pulled out the tie to replace it in the box. He locked it in the bottom desk drawer.

It was at the last departmental luncheon before the conference when he had truly lost it. The usual departmental politics was at play. Nothing unusual. But he lashed out at colleagues. He bullied young assistants. He made enemies. The disease and its treatment held him underwater. He scrambled for a toehold on the steeply slanting floor of the pool.

A young associate professor was trying to gain points. Some part of Jeffrey understood. He had done the same thing in his climb to department head. She brought up a well-researched and clever subject for the conference. She didn't know.

"I think it's a great idea to have a panel on

developmental and pathological gynecomastia."

The other people at lunch looked down at their plates. She raced on through the awkward silence.

"Gynecomastia. You know, the little breasts men get from being fat or having their hormones out of balance. Older men, uh, and men with extra weight." Jeffrey sucked in his belly while the other diners searched their plates for the last crumbs of comfort.

"The fat cells make estrogen and stimulate breast formation. It can cause breast cancer and make finding breast cancer tumors more difficult to detect. African American men with graduate degrees or in managerial positions are more at risk." Here, she had looked around, confused by the stony silence.

Jeffrey slammed into the bottom of the pool with enough force to push out the last of the air from his lungs. He screamed underwater. An icy stream of polluted cells rushed into his mouth.

His true enemy in the department, the good old boy who wanted his position, had chimed in, "Such an irony that men should have to deal with a female illness."

Jeffrey had grasped the table. His brown knuckles had strained white against the wood. He yelled, "Enough. Stop talking. Stop talking. I don't have breast cancer." He smacked the table hard enough to drive a splinter deep into his palm. Diners throughout the restaurant turned to watch him lose control.

He couldn't stop.

"Drop the whole subject, this lying pile of shit everyone is feeding me." Jeffrey felt his blood pressure skyrocket.

One of his female colleagues began to cry. Jeffrey had a moment of shame for his behavior but his fury over everything rose up again.

"I'm going. You sort out the precious conference. You think I don't know what is going on but I do. You're trying to make me out to be sick but you're the ones who are sick. I run this department. You want to take over my position but you can't have it. You work for me." He had ranted at the top of his lungs, calling them gutless and mealy-mouthed before stumbling out of the restaurant. All collegiate grace and agility shed.

In the blinding light on the street, the fatigue rolled over him. With it came shame, embarrassment, and the acknowledgement of loss.

Alone in his office, Jeffrey sat with the heels of his hands digging into his cheeks. Unlocking the desk drawer, he took a pair of sharp scissors and cut the pink tie to ribbons. While one hand gathered together the fragments into a pile, the fingers of his other hand probed at the wound of his tumor. He worried the lumpectomy scar. Gently he traced the edges of the radiation burns over and over again until he came to know his place. A body punctured and burned. No longer a man. At the mercy of other people for the first time in many years. Dependent on their good will. With only a diagnosis as an identity.

Jeffrey let out a deep breath, feeling the pull of the scar and the tearing of the irradiated area. With a swipe, the desecrated pink fabric scuttled over the desk to float in an untidy mess towards the waiting trashcan. Breaking the water's surface to gulp air, he dialed a number.

"Daniel, this is Jeffrey."

Malignancy

One in two men will be diagnosed with cancer in their lifetime. One of every hundred patients treated for breast cancer is a man. Men are more likely to die of prostate and pancreatic cancer than breast cancer but an estimated 410 American men died of breast cancer in 2012 with 2190 new cases of male breast cancer diagnosed that year. Researchers note an increase in the rate of breast cancer in men but have difficulty making predictions due to the relatively small number of cases available to study. In India, 0.7% of all new cancer diagnoses in men are classified as breast cancer. Breast cancer is diagnosed most often in men between the ages of 60 and 70 with an average age of 67 in the US. American men and women have similar survival rates at five and ten years.

Risk factors for male breast cancer are similar to the risk factors for female breast cancer. Factors include exposure to female hormones (estrogen and progesterone – from changing hormone levels and from medications to treat other illnesses), obesity, and BRCA mutation carriers. BRCA mutations can be passed through male and female relatives. Liver disease, chronic alcoholism and Klinefelter's Syndrome are known risk factors for men. Trauma to the breast is being investigated as a risk factor for breast cancer development. A study is following male soldiers in Germany who grew a left breast. This study suggests asymmetrical gynecomastia develops from repeated trauma (thumping a rifle against the left chest) that stimulated the growth of left breast tissue.

Breast cancer in men can metastasize or spread faster due to the closeness of the male breast to skin, nipple, and muscle tissue. Breast cancer in men can metastasize to lungs, liver, bones, and brain. Like female cases, breast cancer travels through the lymphatic system and the blood stream.

While lesions may be easier to feel on a man's chest, gynecomastia (the development of male breasts) and men's lack of awareness may inhibit them from detecting changes in their breasts as early on as women find changes. Usually male breast cancer is found at a more advanced state, Stage III or State IV where it has spread beyond the breast tissue into the lymph nodes or into other organs and tissues. Like women, mammography, ultrasound, needle biopsy and excisional biopsy are used to diagnosis breast cancer in men.

Male breast cancer is treated with the same protocols as breast cancer in postmenopausal women. Treatment methods include mastectomy, lumpectomy, chemotherapy, and radiation or some combination of the methods. Most males will receive hormonal therapy that can lead to hot flashes and impotence. The United Kingdom is publishing preliminary papers exploring biological differences between male and female breast cancers. This information will have implications for different diagnosis and treatment protocols in men and women.

An important area to be studied is the unequal statistics for male breast cancer across different American racial categories. Breast cancer is usually diagnosed in African American males between ages 60 and 70 but it is most often diagnosed in African American men who are college graduates and in professional or managerial roles. African American males are 49% less likely to be referred to a medical oncologist and 56% less likely to receive chemotherapy than White American males. African American men have a 66% survival rate from breast cancer compared to the 90% survival rate of the White males diagnosed with breast cancer. The death rate from breast cancer in African American men is 33% higher than in African American women diagnosed with breast cancer.

References:

Administration, Breast Cancer Campaign. "Differences Found between Male and Female Breast Cancers." *Research that Saves Lives*. Breast Cancer Campaign, 24 Nov. 2011. Web. 29 Jan. 2013. <http://www.breastcancercampaign.org/articles/differences-found-between-male-and-female-breast-cancers>.

Anderson, William F., Ismail Jatoi, Julia Tse, and Philip S. Rosenber. "Male Breast Cancer: A Population-Based Comparison with Female Breast Cancer." *Journal of Clinical Oncology* 28.2 (2010): 232-239. Print.

"Breast Cancer in Men." *Breast Cancer Health Center*. Web MD, n.d. Web. 18 May 2013. <http://www.webmd.com/breast-cancer/guide/breast-cancer-men>.

Brooks, Megan. "An Equalizer for One Racial Disparity in Breast Cancer." *Medscape Multispecialty*. Medscape Medical News, 3 Oct. 2012. Web. 30 Dec. 2012. <http://www.medscape.com/viewarticle/772016>.

"Cancer Advances: Racial Differences Seen in Male Breast Cancer Survival." *Cancer.Net*. American Society of Clinical Oncology, 20 Mar. 2007. Web. 30 Sept. 2013. <http://www.cancer.net/cancer-advances-racial-differences-seen-male-breast-cancer-survival>.

Conrad Stoppler, Melissa. "Male Breast Cancer." *MedicineNet*. Ed. Dennis Lee, and William C. Shiel, Jr.. MedicineNet, 2011. Web. 29 Oct. 2013. <http://www.medicinenet.com/male_breast_cancer/article.htm>.

Crew, Katherine D., Alfred I. Neugut, Xiaoyan Wang, Judith S. Jacobson, Victor R. Grann, George Raptis, and Dawn L. Hershman. "Racial Disparities in Treatment and Survival of Male Breast Cancer." *Journal of Clinical Oncology* 25.9 (2007): 1089-1098. Web. 29 Jan. 2013. <http://jco.ascopubs.org/content/25/9/1089.full>.

Hines, Stephanie L., Mona Yasrebi, Winston W. Tan, Edith A. Perez, and Elizabeth R. DePeri. "The Role of Mammography in Male Patients with Breast Cancer." *Mayo Clinic Proceedings* 82.3 (2007): 297-300. *Elsevier*. Web. 27 Nov. 2013. <http://www.mayoclinicproceedings.org/article/S0025-6196(11)61025-2/abstract>.

"Hormonal Therapy for Male Breast Cancer." *Treatment of Male Breast Cancer*. BreastCancer.org, 17 Sept. 2012. Web. 18 May 2013. <http://www.breastcancer.org/symptoms/types/male_bc/treatment/hormonal>.

Lallanilla, Marc. "Atten-TION: Male Soldiers are Growing Breasts." *Livescience: Strange News*. TechMedia Network, 25 Jan. 2013. Web. 29 Jan. 2013. <http://www.livescience.com/26597-german-army-soldiers-breasts.html>.

"Male Breast Cancer." *Wikipedia: The Free Encyclopedia*. Wikimedia Foundation, Inc., 2012. *http://en.wikipedia.org/wiki/Male_breast_cancer*. Web. 21 Jan. 2013.

Male Breast Cancer Treatment. National Cancer Institute: National Institutes of Health, 2013. *Cancer.gov*. Web. 18 May 2013. <http://www.cancer.gov/cancertopics/pdq/treatment/malebreast/HealthProfessional>.

Mayo Clinic Staff. "Male Breast Cancer." *Health Information*. Mayo Clinic, 13 July 2013. Web. 30 Oct. 2013. <http://www.mayoclinic.com/health/male-breast-cancer/DS00661>.

Mayo Clinic staff. "Male Breast Cancer: Tests and Diagnosis." *Mayo Clinic: Health Information*. Mayo Foundation for Medical Education and Research, 13 July 2013. Web. 27 Nov. 2013. <http://www.mayoclinic.com/health/male-breast-cancer/DS00661/DSECTION=tests-and-diagnosis>.

"Pink Pearls of Hope: Breast Cancer Organization: Special Populations." *Black Onyx - Male Breast Cancer.* Pink Pearls of Hope, n.d. Web. 31 Oct. 2013. <http://www.hopeagainstbc.org/special-populations/black-onyx-male-breast-cancer/>.

Ruddy, K J., and E. P. Winer. "Male Breast Cancer: Risk Factors, Biology, Diagnosis, Treatment , and Survivorship." *Medical Oncology* 24 (2013): 1434-1443. Web. 30 Oct. 2013. <http://annonc.oxfordjournals.org/content/24/6/1434.full.pdf+html>.

"What Are the Key Statistics About Breast Cancer in Men?" *Breast Cancer in Men: Learn about Cancer.* American Cancer Society, 30 Sept. 2013. Web. 30 Oct. 2013. <http://www.cancer.org/cancer/breastcancerinmen/detailedguide/breast-cancer-in-men-key-statistics>.

"What is Gynecomastia?" *Gynecomastia in Men.* Gynecomastia.org, n.d. Web. 26 Jan. 2013. <http://www.gynecomastia.org/gynecomastia-men>.

Yost, Merle. "Gynecomastia and Its Psychological Impact." *Gynecomastia: The Web's Best Resource for Information.* Gynecomastia.org, n.d. Web. 21 Jan. 2013. <http://www.gynecomastia.org/gynecomastia-men/living-gynecomastia/gynecomastia-and-its-psychological-impact>.

Activity1

Go to an office where mammograms are filmed. How are the waiting rooms and offices decorated? What colors are used on the walls, on the paper dressing gowns, on the furniture? What magazines are in the waiting room? What pictures are on the wall?

    Design a waiting room for men.

    Design an exam room for men.

    Design an office for a doctor explaining mammogram results to men.

Would the two offices (the one you explored and the one you would design) be different? Why? Could it impact outcomes of follow through, anxiety/distress, comfort with diagnostic accuracy, compliance/interaction with the treatment protocols, and trust in their doctor's alliance with them?

Activity 2

Role-play 1: A male role-plays the patient. A female role-plays the doctor. The doctor is to tell the patient he has breast cancer and will need follow-up, starting with a visit to a breast surgeon.

Role-play 2: A male role-plays the patient. A male role-plays the doctor. The doctor is to tell the patient he has breast cancer and will need follow-up, starting with a visit to a breast surgeon.

Role-Play 3: A male patient tells his wife he has breast cancer.

Role-Play 4: A male patient tells his male colleague he has breast cancer.

Does gender in the role-play scenarios make a difference in how the information is given? The length of the interaction? The vulnerability of the patient? Would you treat a man different from a woman when giving a diagnosis for breast cancer?
What would happen if the patient was a transgendered individual?

Activity 3

Collect pamphlets about diagnostic screen for breast cancer and treatment protocols for breast cancer (can be found in most mammography and breast surgeon offices or online). Design a pamphlet for men needing diagnostic screening breast cancer protocols such as a needle biopsy or lumpectomy.

What colors, symbols, and resources would you use? Design a pamphlet for men needing treatment for breast cancer including mastectomy, lumpectomy, chemotherapy, radiation, and hormone treatment.

What colors, symbols, and resources would you use? How are the pamphlets different from what you found for women in word choice, symbols, images, and other variables?

Resources:

"Breast Cancer in Men." *Breast Cancer Health Center.* Web MD, n.d. Web. 18 May 2013. <http://www.webmd.com/breast-cancer/guide/breast-cancer-men>.

www.gynecomastia.com (website focused on the male breasts and male breast health with substantial listings of resources)

"Pink Pearls of Hope: Breast Cancer Organization: Special Populations." *Black Onyx - Male Breast Cancer.* Pink Pearls of Hope, n.d. Web. 31 Oct. 2013. <http://www.hopeagainstbc.org/special-populations/black-onyx-male-breast-cancer/>.

Trudi Young Taylor, Ph.D., is a nationally certified and state licensed counselor with over 20 years experience with individual, couple, and group therapy. She has taught in university and community college systems and has designed educational programs for classrooms and communities. With certification and extensive experience in massage therapy and yoga teaching, she integrates her understanding of bodily expression of the human experience into every component of her work. Her short stories have been published in anthologies and online. Breasts Don't Lie is her first collection of short stories.

She welcomes your comments on her website, trudiyoungtaylor.com, and the Breasts Don't Lie FaceBook page.